Housing and Social Services
for the Elderly

Elizabeth D. Huttman
with a chapter by Ilse J. Volinn

The Praeger Special Studies program—utilizing the most modern and efficient book production techniques and a selective worldwide distribution network—makes available to the academic, government, and business communities significant, timely research in U.S. and international economic, social, and political development.

Housing and Social Services for the Elderly

Social Policy Trends

PRAEGER SPECIAL STUDIES IN U.S. ECONOMIC, SOCIAL, AND POLITICAL ISSUES

Praeger Publishers   New York   London

Library of Congress Cataloging in Publication Data

Huttman, Elizabeth D   1929-
   Housing and social services for the elderly.

   (Praeger special studies in U.S. economic, social,
and political issues)
   Includes bibliographical references and index.
   1. Aged—United States—Dwellings.   2. Old age
homes—United States.   3. Aged—Care and hygiene.
4. Social work with the aged—United States.
I. Volinn, Ilse J.   II. Title.
HD7287.92.U54H87   361.6'0973   75-44932
ISBN 0-275-23830-X

PRAEGER PUBLISHERS
383 Madison Avenue, New York, N.Y. 10017, U.S.A.

Published in the United States of America in 1977
by Praeger Publishers,
A Division of Holt, Rinehart and Winston, CBS, Inc.

9   038   9876543

Dedicated to
Anna Jones Dickerson, Who Provided Early
Inspiration to Undertake an Academic Career
and to
the Late Ruth Perren, Zermatt, Who Provided over the
Years a Quiet Mountain Retreat in Which to Design the
Original Study, Write the Original Report, and Write This Book

PREFACE

Since the 1960s, the number of people aged 65 and over has greatly increased. In addition, the proportion living to age 80 has grown so that we are now talking about "young" elderly and "older" elderly. A major concern of these elderly is housing; a major fear is not to be able to any longer stay in one's own home or to continue an independent life style. Above all, it is a concern about keeping out of nursing homes. We share this concern and, as sociologists, firmly believe provision of social services and housing subsidies will greatly enhance the elderly's chances of living the independent life they desire.

This book is written for policy makers, for students of policy issues, and for academics in this field. The purpose has been to try to bring together in one book information and research findings on all aspects of housing the elderly. A chapter has been devoted to types of assistance to the elderly in their own home, and then several chapters to specially designed housing for the elderly. This is followed by a final chapter by Ilse J. Volinn on the nursing home, including a description of the facilities, the funding, the staff, and the patients. In writing this, Dr. Volinn draws on findings from her studies of nursing homes and from major gerontological surveys she directed in the State of Washington. As research director of a statewide health manpower project she was responsible for the gathering and analysis of a wide range of data relative to health care professionals. She has published her research findings in the fields of gerontology, health facilities and health occupations. In her chapter on nursing homes she combines her own data with those of other sources.

In writing the other parts of this book, I have backed up my statements with findings from my nationwide study on subsidized specially designed apartments and congregate housing in Canada. This study included a mailed survey of 294 managers in a sample described in the Appendix; it included interviews with 303 elderly living in 19 such developments; it also included case studies of these 19 developments. As chief investigator, I designed the research instruments, developed the sampling plan, compiled the code book, constructed tables, directed the data processing, analyzed the data, and wrote the report on the user and manager surveys. Douglas Halverson was overall research assistant on this project, and Janet Lee Tse worked with the author. Marie Seto helped with the Vancouver case studies. Michael Audain was overall coordinator for the Canadian Council for Social Development, the sponsoring agency.

In writing this book, the author wishes to acknowledge Douglas Halverson's work on the original Canadian research and especially the Summerset Court case study. She also appreciates the advice of Lucy Bookbinder, who has long been involved with Section 236 housing, Effie Robinson of the Community Services Division of the San Francisco Housing Authority, and Mary James of the Santa Clara County Housing Authority. In regard to the case studies, she especially wants to thank Hal Foster, Ned Holmgren, and Clara Swearington. She wishes to thank Sandra and Dorothy Schwab for the typing, and, last of all, John Huttman for his considerable patience.

Dr. Volinn wishes to thank, for continuous assistance in locating governmental resources and publications, Leocadia Codispoti, Librarian, Northwest Federal Regional Council Library, Region X, Department of Health, Education and Welfare, Seattle; for her valuable comments and generous sharing of a wealth of experience, Ruth M. Ward, Region X Office of Aging, Office of Human Development, Department of Health, Education and Welfare, Seattle; and Alma M. Ware, Assistant Professor in Physiological Nursing, School of Nursing, University of Washington, Seattle, who contributed valuable suggestions to the section on nursing care and its criteria, and made many resources available.

CONTENTS

LIST OF TABLES

Housing and Social Services for the Elderly

CHARACTERISTICS OF
THE ELDERLY

This book describes the various social policy alternatives for housing the elderly and the social services necessary to increase the ability of the elderly to fully enjoy their housing. The basic assumption that underlies all the material in this book is that the elderly have certain characteristics and, related to these, certain physical, economic, psychological, and social limitations that must be taken into account in meeting their housing needs. In other words, the elderly's requirements in the housing area are different from those of families and, moreover, extend beyond simply providing adequate shelter. A second assumption is that many elderly can continue to live an independent life if these housing and service needs are fully met, where otherwise many of them will have to prematurely go into a nursing home or another institutional setting. Researchers have calculated that one-third or more of those in nursing homes might be able to use alternative, less intensive, care facilities like congregate housing if such existed.[1] Many counselors of senior citizens give us examples of how the elderly might have stayed in their own home if supportive services could have taken care of certain needs.

These needs will vary and thus the type of housing considered most suitable will vary, for within the U.S. elderly population of 22.4 million (1972) are many subgroups with different physical, economic, and psychological limitations. Any social policy recommendations must take into account these variations and suggest a variety of alternatives. No one course will fit the needs of all elderly. Thus different chapters of this book are devoted to describing housing alternatives, including living in one's own home, in specially designed elderly apartment complexes, in nursing homes. The effort here is, first, to bring together in one book material on the many different housing alternatives so as to allow policy makers to see the array available and better evaluate what housing will best fit the needs of what particular elderly population. Second, the material presented will hopefully lead policy makers to fund and promote all the necessary ingredients to make each type of housing adequately serve the population it is meant for, stressing again that needs are more than simply provision of shelter.

In following this theme of provision of more than shelter, we devote an early chapter to describing the services that can be made available and the financial assistance programs that can be useful to those elderly still living in their own home. After this we concentrate on specially designed elderly housing alternatives, with several chapters on facilities and services that should be included in such apartment complexes and on the congregate housing developments that include a dining room and hotel-type bedrooms.

The discussion is based on several research studies the author has conducted on elderly housing. One is a nationwide three-part study of subsidized specially designed housing for the elderly in Canada. First, a survey was conducted of a stratified sample of 294 managers-sponsors of such elderly apartment and congregate developments; second, interviews were held with 303 elderly in 19 developments; third, case studies were done of these 19 developments. In the United States, the author was a consultant on a study of over 1,200 elderly in private housing in eight cities; these elderly were participating in the experimental housing allowance program (HAP) sponsored by the U.S. Department of Housing and Urban Development (HUD). In addition, the author has done a number of case studies of specially designed housing developments in the West and Midwest. (See the Appendix for methodology used in the Canadian study.)

In North America these specially designed elderly developments are increasing in number, due to the insistent efforts of experts in geriatrics and elderly housing who see the need for alternatives to the nursing home. This need has become evident as the extended longevity of the elderly has meant that, out of the 22.4 million aged 65 and over in our population in 1972, many now live into their eighties; thus there are a number who have some degree of physical frailty, psychological limitation, and financial deprivation that makes it hard for them to stay in their own home. Although these elderly are still ambulatory and active and alert enough to maintain an independent or semi-independent life, they may have trouble with cooking, shopping, housekeeping, or exterior maintenance of their home. As their own energies and resources become inadequate to cope with daily demands of living, due to the aging process, provision of adequate alternative housing is needed that can allow them to maintain an active life and to prevent them from moving to the role of dependence and loss of functioning in an institutional setting. Specially designed individual apartments and congregate living arrangements can provide this environment for independent or semiindependent living.

Before any of these housing arrangements are discussed, it is necessary to give some idea of the characteristics and conditions of the elderly, as these conditions will influence the types of provisions we make for serving their housing and social service needs. In doing so, it is hoped we create an awareness of the many subgroups that exist among the elderly and a realization that instead of one housing policy direction for all elderly, we need a number of alternative policies. Like the rest of us, the elderly include a variety of types of citizens in the United States, from the rich to the poor, black to white, upper class to lower class, and conservative to liberal. They have a variety of life styles and ways of looking at the world. They want different things, with some preferring to be in retirement communities and others with their families; some wanting privacy and little interaction and others wanting to be near children or interact in leisure activities. As one 81-year-old Gray Panther woman said: "We're just like everyone else but older. We want to be seen as individuals."

While keeping this in mind, there are certain generalizations that are useful in dealing with the elderly and ascertaining, hopefully with the elderly themselves, their need priorities. A basic fact is that the elderly in the United States made up over 10 percent of our population and 19 percent of the households in 1970,[2] and, as the U.S. birthrate goes down, they proportionately become more important. Within this elderly group, the fastest growing subgroup is the group 80 and over, followed by the 70–80-year-old group, a fact that greatly influences the type of housing needed.

NUMBER OF ELDERLY

In 1960 there were 5.6 million persons 75 and over, while by 1970 there were 7.6 million. Between 1960 and 1970 the rate of increase for the general population was 13 percent, but for the whole elderly population it was 21 percent and for the population 75 and over it was even greater. At present about 40 percent of the elderly are 75 and over, while 7 percent of them are actually 85 and over.[3]

The sheer number of elderly in the United States today is a fact that must be kept in mind even more than their proportion in the population. The 22.4 million aged 65 and over in the United States in 1972 equaled the population of many medium–sized countries. Further, we had almost one and a half million elderly aged 85 and over, and therefore a rather large population of people that had very special needs, both medical and housing.

Geographical Distribution

These elderly are not evenly distributed throughout the United States. They are more likely to be found in both rural areas and central city areas. Over one-fourth of those 65 and over are located in rural areas and another third are in central city areas. A much smaller group, only a fifth, are residing in suburban or urban fringe areas.[4] However, as U.S. postwar suburban settlers have begun to age, their representation in the suburban population has been increasing, from 16.5 percent in 1960 to 21.2 percent in 1970.[5] At present the low concentration of these elderly in the suburbs and the low density of the elderly population in rural areas, plus their lower income, make it hard to provide needed services to these groups; in contrast, the high concentration of elderly in certain central city areas facilitates the provision of an array of services.

The elderly also are concentrated in certain states and cities, with Florida leading, with 12 percent of its population elderly; in many of its cities, such as Miami Beach, St. Petersburg, Port Charlotte, elderly represent as much as 30 percent of the population. States with 11.6 percent or more of their population elderly in 1970 were the sparsely populated, mainly rural states of Maine, South Dakota, Iowa, Nebraska, and Missouri. In contrast, Alaska, Nevada, Utah, New Mexico, Virginia, and South Carolina had less than 7.6 percent of their population elderly.[6]

There is another type of maldistribution of the elderly population: females outnumber males, with 72.8 males for every 100 females in the elderly population in 1970. As age increases, this becomes more apparent, with a very large percentage of the elderly over 75 being female.[7] This of course means there are many widows in the elderly population. In 1970, almost a third of the entire elderly population was composed of widowed women, in total about six million women. Looked at another way, 52 percent of the total female elderly population were widowed, and by age 80, over 72 percent were widowed. Many of these women have, for most of their adult life, been financially and psychologically dependent on their husbands; a number of them now find it hard to deal with financial and legal problems or to adjust to living alone.

Elderly men, in contrast to the women, are usually married, with only 17.1 percent widowed; even of elderly men aged 80-84, only 32 percent were widowed.[9]

On the other hand, when looking at the marital status of the elderly, one must point out almost half in 1970 were married and living with their husbands or wives; of course, this was truer of those in the age group 65-74.[10]

Race and Ethnicity

The elderly population has an overrepresentation of foreign born, with 15 percent of the elderly, compared to 5 percent of the total population, in 1970 foreign born. In this elderly population there is, however, an underrepresentation of blacks, with only 8 percent of the elderly population black, compared to 11 percent of the total population.[11] The underrepresentation of blacks among the elderly is due to the higher death rate of blacks in the past; this is beginning to change. However, even with an underrepresentation in 1970, there were almost 1.6 million black elderly; and this particular group was in special need of housing, because, compared to white elderly, there were more of them proportionately in substandard units, and more living in rental housing. Moreover, statistics show few black elderly are to be found in private intermediate care facilities and nursing homes, although they are well-represented in public housing.

Living Arrangements: Proximity of Family

The major fact to keep in mind is that 28 percent of the elderly live alone; twice as many elderly women live alone as men, indicating a number of isolated widows who may lack needed services. Only 4.8 percent of the elderly live in institutions and only 0.7 percent in boardinghouses or other group quarters.[12]

In evaluating the situation of those living alone, one must assess how well their family can still cover their needs. Family proximity is one measure. Ethel Shanas found in one study that, of the elderly who had children, 56 percent lived within one hour's drive of them and only 16 percent lived more than an hour away; 28 percent of elderly lived with their adult children.[13] In our Canadian interviews with elderly residents of specially designed housing, we found a number of the elderly residents of these apartment and congregate developments did not have children in the area; 44 percent had no children alive or none living in the immediate area; 33 percent had neither children nor other relatives in the area (see Table 1.1). However, of those that did have children in the area, 87 percent had daily or weekly contact, either by visit or by phone.[14]

Income

One of the main problems many elderly have is lack of a sufficient income to meet daily needs. Almost half (47 percent) of the elderly households in 1970 had incomes of $3,000 or less; half of these support families on less than $1,000 a year. One out of four elderly

persons is poor. Elderly persons living alone were even more likely
to be existing below the poverty level in 1970, with 53.5 percent of
such women and 43.4 percent of such men living alone being at or below the poverty level. [15]

The average annual income of the elderly is far below that of
the general population; in 1970 for all men it was $7,426 while for
men 65 and over it was $4,550; for all women it was $3,156 but for
elderly women it was $2,214 (see Table 1.2). Since two-thirds of the
elderly men had wives to support, their situation was not that much
better than that of the women. The annual income went down drastically both for men and women as their age increased, with men making
at least $1,500 less when they were 75 and over than when they were
65-69. Women and blacks 75 and over did even worse, with women
in this group having a median annual income of $1,335, black women
having $974, and black men, $1,503. In general, only 14 percent of
all elderly had incomes of $10,000 and over, thus indicating a small
group that could afford Leisure World or a similar retirement facility. [16]
As Shanas has pointed out, median retirement incomes are often far
below what is needed to keep up former life styles. The elderly have
the dilemma of wanting to continue to occupy the same house they
lived in when their incomes were higher. [17] Yet, even if they completely paid off the mortgage on the house, as 82 percent of the 8.4

TABLE 1.1

Elderly Persons with Children Living and in Area, by Development
Type

Development Type	None Living or None in Area	Some in Area	No Answer	Total
All				
Number	132	170	1	303
Percent	43.6	56.1	0.3	100
Self-contained apartments				
Number	44	72	0	116
Percent	37.9	62.1	0.0	100
All congregate and mixed				
Number	88	98	1	187
Percent	47.1	52.4	0.5	100

Source: Canadian user survey.

TABLE 1.2

Incomes of Families and Individuals: 1970
(median income in dollars)

Income Group	Families	Percent in United States	Indi- viduals	Percent in United States
U.S. average	9,867	100	3,137	100
Family head/indi- vidual, 65 years of age and over				
All races	5,053	51	1,951	62
White	5,263	53	2,005	64
Black	3,282	33	1,443	46

Source: U.S. Bureau of the Census, Current Population Reports (Washington, D.C.: U.S. Government Printing Office).

million elderly household owners in 1970 had,[18] they are faced with the worry of meeting the increasingly high taxes. Many of these homeowners are near or below the poverty level—39 percent, in 1970[19] (see Table 1.3).

Furthermore, in most cases the home is the elderly person's only financial asset, though its median value in 1970 was only $14,000 for all areas and about $15,000 for central city areas.[20] These elderly are continually confronted with the need to turn this asset into liquid funds. One large study of the assets of the elderly in 1967 found the median amount of financial assets at that time for all elderly households was $542. For those with incomes of $2,000–2,999, assets were $900, while they were far less for those with lower incomes, and in fact zero for about a fifth of the total elderly surveyed. However, assets ran $10,000 and over for the group of elderly with incomes of $7,500 of more,[21] again showing the variety of incomes and savings in this 22.4–million population group. Under 30 percent of the 1970 population 65 and over got any income from wages and salaries or self-employment; * 45 percent got some income from assets, though it was usually low; most got social security and around 12 percent got

---

*The 1970 census data show even less participation in the civilian labor force, only 16.6 percent for all elderly 65 and over, though 25.2 percent for all males, compared to 10.2 percent for all females.

what was then old-age assistance (OAA) and is now supplementary
security income (SSI), according to the Facts on Aging report of the
U.S. Department of Health, Education and Welfare (HEW). Others
got railroad retirement money, veterans' benefits (12 percent), government employees' retirement benefits (8 percent), or private pensions (12 percent).[22]

Health Status of the Elderly

Physical or biological changes are part of the aging process.
These, however, can be different from chronological age, for the
functioning of the physical organism is not the same for everyone
aged 65 or 75. There are several kinds of physiological processes
that generally decline with age, but individual characteristics may
cause the decline to be fast for one person and slow in another. Thus
one person aged 75 may be in a nursing home suffering from senility
and heart disease while another person is actively playing golf and
keeping his or her own home. Fred Cottrell explains this biological
process by saying:

> There are only a few of the characteristics of older people
> that are universal among them. Of the traits that they do
> share, not all show up at the same age in all older people.
> Senescence is a catch all word that is often used when no
> other more specific one, like blindness, arteriosclerosis,
> aging, or arthritis, will fit. In another sense, it covers
> all of the adverse conditions that accompany old age. In
> still another, it means only the results of "normal" aging.
> In this sense, senescence characterizes everybody who
> lives long enough. In time, the skin gets wrinkled, mottled,
> and while easily broken, heals slowly. Appetite fails and
> weight is often reduced. Muscle tone declines. Usually
> one or more of the senses declines in sensitivity. Sexual
> vigor is reduced.
>   Another combination of less easily observable symp-
> toms can be discovered by use of instruments like the
> stethoscope. . . . Blood chemistry show definite changes
> that are characteristic of the aged. But almost every one
> of these symptoms also occurs in greater or lesser degree
> among people who are not called senescent or senile.[23]

Margaret Hellie Huyck, in Growing Older, points out that physical capacity and physical functioning decrease as one ages, just as
Cottrell has noted in the statement above.[24] She says a person's or-

TABLE 1.3

Socioeconomic and Housing Characteristics of the Elderly
(persons 65 years and over, in thousands)

Living Arrangement	Number	Percent
In housing units	18,994	94.5
Owned units	13,591	67.6
Rented units	5,403	26.9
In group quarters	1,107	5.5
Nursing homes and homes for aged	924	4.6
Other quarters	183	0.9
Total	20,101	100
In housing units		
With all plumbing	17,480	92.0
Lacking plumbing	1,514	8.0
Total	18,994	100
Not crowded	18,517	97.0
Overcrowded	477	3.0
Total	18,994	100

Source: U.S. Department of Commerce, Bureau of the Census, Subject Report: Housing of Senior Citizens, 1970 (Washington, D.C.: U.S. Government Printing Office, 1972).

gans diminish in function over time. For example, a person has, on the average, only 92 percent of his former brain weight when he is 75, compared to when he was 30; he has only 84 percent of his basal metabolism rate and 70 percent of his breathing capacity.[25] The body burns up food less efficiently than when younger and the excess turns to fat. Exertion is harder, taking more energy outlay, a fact one needs to remember in designing housing for the elderly. Fat replaces some of the heart muscles, thus meaning the heart does not always get the proper amounts of oxygenated blood. This can cause breathlessness and coldness in the feet and hands, a fact that one should keep in mind in heating elderly housing. The veins and the arteries may be clogged, with fatty cells doing the clogging.

Changes in nerve cells cause slower response. By age 70, one usually has 20 or so percent less neurons present than at birth, because the nerve cells have died or been destroyed. Because neurons conduct "information" or sensory impulses to the muscles, the brain, and other tissues, there can be a slower response and slower movement, a situation that needs to be recognized in provision of services to the elderly.[26]

With advanced age the sensory system deteriorates. One has a decrease in the senses of smell, sight, and hearing, all factors affecting housing design.[27]

There is also a reduced capacity for the body to recover from stress. Change can be viewed as stressful and can make an elderly person physically or emotionally sick. For example, the high death rate of widows and widowers in the first year after a spouse's death is contributed to by the stress of this event or change.[28]

All these facts show up in the statistics on the health of the elderly, such as those from the National Health Survey. Over 40 percent of U.S. elderly in 1970, the national survey showed, had some "activity limitation" caused by a chronic condition; 20 percent were limited in physical mobility, housebound, or bedridden. In this National Health Survey the most common activity limitations were arthritis and rheumatism, and heart condition, with a fifth of those who said they had an activity limitation due to a chronic condition mentioning heart conditions as the problem, and another fifth giving arthritis and rheumatism as the chronic illness; visual impairments were the next most likely mentioned condition.[29]

In the survey (on which the author served as consultant) of an active group of elderly using or applying for housing allowances in eight cities, there were still 17 percent who said they had severe health problems and almost half of the surveyed group said they had at least some health problems; a large proportion had difficulty getting places. Again, heart trouble and arthritis-rheumatism were the main health problems.

In our Canadian survey of 303 elderly living in specially designed apartments and congregate housing, a third said they had physical limitations that caused difficulty in getting around. Interviewers felt 39 percent of their respondents were obviously ill or infirm or somewhat infirm. Again, in the Canadian study, the major problems involved the heart and circulation, with one-third having these problems, arthritis and rheumatism, and eye troubles.[30]

These surveys all give self-evaluations of health conditions by the elderly and thus there may be overemphasis of some illnesses and underreporting of other illnesses. Cope W. Schwenger, in his study of Ontario (Canada) elderly, took a more expensive route to finding the health condition of a small part of his sample, 29 persons in two housing projects: he had a doctor do a physical examination and classify the findings. Again the most prevalent illness was circulatory; a much smaller group had problems of the nervous system and sense organs, followed by a group with problems of bones and organs of movement. For his total sample of almost 600 elderly over 70, about three-fourths had illnesses they mentioned to the interviewer, again indicating that a high proportion of the elderly have some health problem.[31]

E. Pfeiffer verifies this in his community study of health conditions of the elderly; he found evidence of "significant" impairment (that is, moderate to complete) for an overall total of 41 percent of his surveyed older citizens, when he included economic, social, and self-care functioning.[32] L. Gottesman, M. Moss, and F. Worts, in their Philadelphis Geriatric Center local surveys, put the figure at over 25 percent.[33] In Shanas' studies she showed that one-fourth of all persons 65 and over who lived in the community needed home care services.[34] To all these studies we must add another proportion of the elderly—5 percent—who are already getting health care in institutions.

PHYSICAL, PSYCHOLOGICAL, ECONOMIC, AND SOCIAL LIMITATIONS

Physical Limitations

Because of the health problems mentioned above, many elderly have physical limitations of various types that affect housing design and services.

Reduced energy is one limitation that must be taken into consideration in designing the interior of special units for the elderly; their low degree of physical exertion means doors must be easy to open, cupboards easy to reach, and rest places made available. Reduced energy may mean that if the elderly are to stay in their existing housing they need help with maintenance and even housework. However, reduced energy may instead mean they need to move to alternative specially designed elderly units because they have difficulty doing maintenance or housework or cooking. In our Canadian study of those in specially designed housing, we found a number moved to these special units specifically because they could no longer perform these tasks; a third of the surveyed Canadian elderly had difficulty with housework and over a fifth had trouble with cooking. Many found maintenance of a house now too much for them.[35]

Problems caused by a deteriorated sensory system, such as those related to seeing, hearing, and smelling, and to poor circulation and resulting coldness, may also mean that elderly need extra provisions in their present home, such as a better heating system, or that they need to move to housing designed to meet these needs.

Health conditions, causing slow movement as well as decreased energy, result in mobility problems for the elderly (see Table 1.4). If a person is to stay in his home, it means that either services must be brought to him, as he or she does not have the mobility to travel to such services, or he must live where services are nearby. The mobility of the elderly person therefore restricts his locational choice.

In building specially designed elderly housing, it means the development must be sited close to needed services such as grocery store, medical centers, and recreational facilities. Siting or locating a development in an outer area, inaccessible to services, is usually not advisable. However, this may depend on availability of transportation.

The mobility problem means more attention must be paid to public transportation. Due to physical limitations, many elderly no longer drive automobiles or no longer can walk long distances to a bus stop or to services. Therefore, there has to be a concern about the availability of special transportation services or the closeness of the bus stop, with the latter influencing the siting of the project (see Table 1.5).

These physical limitations and the resulting immobility can inhibit social interaction. To counteract this, outreach services must be extended to elderly still in their own home. In the case of designing special elderly housing, layout and facilities must be so planned to stimulate interaction.

Health problems that cause a person to require medication, a special diet, or walking aids mean that nursing or homemaker services must be provided in the person's home or apartment. Congregate housing with special nursing services may be required if the person is to avoid a nursing home.

However, health problems may mean the elderly person is reluctant to move out of his present dwelling unit. The exertion both for the search for housing and for the move to this housing is considered too much. Therefore the person neither goes to specially designed elderly housing, nor uses a housing allowance program, if such exists, to move to a standard private unit. The loss of energy as well as fear may also mean the person is reluctant to move from one level of specially designed housing to a higher level, such as congregate housing, even though his health situation has deteriorated. This is a problem existing in many public housing projects. As the chief public housing spokesman for the Canadian province of Ontario pointed out in regard to occupants of their 18,000 elderly housing units:

TABLE 1.4

Outdoor Activity, by Health Status

Health Status	Not Daily or Irregular	Daily Less Than One Hour (and maybe less in winter)	Daily One Hour or More, or Daily One Hour and More (except possibly in winter)	No Answer	Total
Seriously limited ability					
Number	11	4	0	0	15
Percent	73.3	26.7	0	0	100
Moderately limited ability					
Number	27	10	15	1	53
Percent	50.9	18.9	28.3	1.9	100
Slightly limited ability					
Number	44	31	33	0	108
Percent	40.7	28.7	30.6	0	100
No incapacity					
Number	15	25	87	0	127
Percent	11.8	19.7	68.5	0	100
Total					
Number	97	70	135	1	303
Percent	32.0	23.2	44.5	0.3	100

Source: Canadian user study.

13

TABLE 1.5

Local Travel Ease, by Development Type

| | Development Type | | |
Travel Ease	Self-Contained Apartments	Congregate with Some Self-Contained Apartments	All
Difficulty getting places			
Number	28	62	90
Percent	24.1	33.1	29.7
No difficulty			
Number	86	104	190
Percent	74.1	55.5	62.7
Does not go out			
Number	2	19	21
Percent	1.8	10.1	6.9
No answer			
Number	0	2	2
Percent	0.0	1.3	0.7
Total			
Number	116	187	303
Percent	100	100	100

Source: Canadian user study.

> From our experience with existing senior citizen projects,
> there is every indication that tenants will stay in these self-
> contained units until death or severe disability occurs . . .
> we must gear ourselves to better serve the older age
> group in our early projects, with its changing physical, so-
> cial and psychological needs. In effect we must broaden
> our services at both ends of the senior spectrum—and
> often within the same building.[36]

This situation of the longevity of residents in elderly housing projects
is indeed a cause for bringing in more services. Marie McGuire
Thompson has long campaigned for such services and facilities and is
one of those responsible for the broadening of allowable facilities in
HUD-sponsored public housing projects.[37]

Psychological Limitations

This reluctance to change living units for more suitable or adequate ones is also due to psychological factors. It is psychologically difficult for the elderly person in his seventies to make a change in his living arrangements; he usually is more set in his habits than a younger person. The elderly person usually has lived in a dwelling unit for many years and it is familiar territory. A move from it can be stressful. An elderly person worries comparatively more about such psychological stresses and suffers actual illness from the stress. Thus he may want to avoid a situation such as a move to another unit.

Data show almost half of the U.S. elderly homeowners have lived in their homes 20 years or more; thus they have strong attachments to this home.[38] Elderly renters also have long-term attachment to one unit. The 1970 census showed only 14 percent of the elderly households, compared to 25 percent of the nonelderly, moved in that year. This may be why so many elderly are concentrated in older inner city areas. Even though the area has deteriorated and the ethnic or racial background of the younger residents has changed, the elderly stay on, for as Paul Niebanck says, among the elderly "there is a tendency to cling as long as possible to the familiar home."[39] For example, in a Model Cities area in Rochester, New York, as reported in The Urban Elderly Poor, almost three-fourths of the elderly whites had lived in their home 16 years or more, even though the area had a sizable black population; only 29 percent of the black elderly had lived in the area that long.[40] The elderly have memories of the neighborhood as it used to be. They have nostalgia for both the neighborhood and the home.

Even when elderly do move, it is often within the same neighborhood, as M. Powell Lawton found.[41] For the elderly the fear of unfamiliar surroundings where stores and services are unknown is great.

The move also means one has to reestablish ties of friendship, and there is not always the willingness or ability to make new friends at the age of 70. At this age, in fact, these persons may depend more on local friendship ties than when they were younger, as Irving Rosow points out. He feels the residential concentration of the elderly encourages friendship ties. In his study of 1,200 elderly in a Cleveland neighborhood, he found where there was a dense population there was more likelihood that the elderly, especially working-class elderly, would have a high degree of contact with each other.[42]

It is no wonder elderly resist the change of area. A Cornell study found 70-80 percent of the surveyed elderly households were unwilling to leave their neighborhood.[43] Relocation studies have found the move so stressful that it may have caused an increased death rate among those who were forced to move.[44]

Moving also means one has to re-create one's personal space, as Huyck points out.[45] This means trying to reduce one's possessions to those most valued and disregarding others. Moving to an elderly project may also mean giving up a sense of separateness and independence and privacy. At an advanced age this privacy is of immense importance to many elderly. In our Canadian survey of elderly residents, the desire for privacy was mentioned often; most did not want to share facilities such as bathroom or sleeping room.

Economic Limitations

Retirement from the work force means a lower income; widowhood may alter economic circumstances even more drastically. At the same time, inflation means costs are going up; health conditions mean medical expenses increase. Thus, severe income deficiencies arise for many elderly, as mentioned above.

These income problems are extreme for the large group of elderly homeowners who want to hold on to a family home, a home that, while it has gone up in market value, is costing more to keep due to increasing taxes and maintenance expenses. To survive, many elderly homeowners simply ignore repairs and thus they often occupy units that in one way or another are below adequate housing standards. These homeowners will also frequently skimp on heating and other utilities or fail to repair broken fixtures, again lowering the quality of the housing they occupy. When these elderly finally do change housing due to cost factors, the change may be to inner city rental units or poorly constructed mobile homes or inadequate structures in rural backwashes, where services are lacking. Moreover, elderly that are long-time residents of remote farmhouses do not move closer to services when health deteriorates, simply because of housing costs.

Economic limitations also mean a number of elderly renters will live in inadequate housing such as transient hotels or prewar apartments in rundown inner city areas. Yet, even in this housing, with inflation the once cheap rents are increasing to beyond the elderly's means. These elderly have a high housing cost burden, with over half of them paying 35 percent or more of their income for rent.[46]

Economic limitations also mean many elderly try to economize on food expenditures in order to pay the rent. The resulting inadequate nutritional intake may lead to health problems. At the same time, these poor elderly may also try to keep down doctor's visits and drug bills, and this in turn has the effect of soon accentuating health problems and making it impossible for these elderly to stay in their own home.

Economic limitations can also mean an elderly person can no longer keep a car or afford a taxi, and thus does not get to needed services or take part in social organizations. Economic limitations can mean that some cannot afford to live in a senior housing development even though such a complex meets their housing needs. Even Section 236 housing (under the U.S. subsidized housing program) may be too expensive for them. If they do get in they have months when they cannot pay the rent or need to apply for the rent supplement. Many Section 236 projects have had numerous vacancies just because many elderly in the local population cannot afford to live in them. The same is true for congregate developments with their dining arrangements; and, if meals are optional in the congregate development, many elderly may not take them simply because they feel they cannot afford them. This situation of limited financial resources of the elderly also means that many congregate developments, to keep the rent low, must house three or four persons to a room.

Social Limitations

Economic and health limitations may mean the elderly person has social adjustments to make. There may be role changes and status changes he or she must now reluctantly face. Today there is institutionalized retirement from employment, accompanied by institutionalized pension pay. Yet the adjustment from a work role to a leisure role is not easy for most in a society that has been strongly dominated by a work ethic. Work took up time, gave one an activity, and provided social contacts and friendships. Work gave one status; a person was identified in terms of being a doctor, a shop owner, a factory supervisor. Life goals, satisfaction, and morale of men have been related to the work setting. Retirement represents for the man discontinuity, a sharp shift in one's role. In fact, some would say there is no clearly defined position or role for the aged in our society; many may not even have an age-related reference group, as Rosow states.[47] The degree to which these elderly are resocialized to this new stage of life may vary; it may relate to how much one associates with other persons of the same age group. Vern L. Bengtson states that overall "the thing to be noted is the prominent lack of institutional provisions—that is, the outer aspects of socialization—to assist the individual in adapting to the marked changes in the social system that are a usual concomitant to growing old."[48] Adapting to change may depend more on a lifetime coping style than on age, R. J. Havighurst, B. L. Neugarten, and others tell us. Havighurst says that a "twenty year series of studies has brought us to the conclusion that personality organization and coping style is the major factor in the life adjustment of the individual as he grows older."[49] Neugarten, while she sees certain personality traits related to age, indicates that "other factors such as work status, health, financial resources, and marital status, are more cogent than chronological age in influencing degrees of adjustment in persons aged 50 and over."[50]

Thus one can say the degree to which role loss and status loss exist may vary. R. A. Atchley's statement that "on the basis of their age, older people usually are relegated to a position in society in which they are no longer judged to be of any use or importance" may apply to many elderly but not to all.[51] As Bengtson says, status in old age may be based more on ascribed than achieved factors.[52] The elderly couple with a large house, still belonging to the local country club, taking cruises, playing golf, may keep their high status even though the man is no longer employed in a high-status occupation. It may be an ascribed status in that it is a status based on his past role.

Besides loss of role, there may be a decrease in the actual number of roles. Bengtson says:

> From research by Havighurst and Albrecht (1953), Maddox 91963), Rosow (1968), Palmore (1968), and others, it seems quite clear that the social world of aging individuals changes, usually contracting with the passage of time. The number and kind of social contacts decreases; roles are literally lost as retirement, widowhood, the death of friends, and decreasing physical mobility leave the individual increasingly to his own resources. This may be viewed as a shrinkage of roles. There is also a general decrease in overall social activity with advancing years.[53]

Bengtson says further that "there are two aspects of role change which affect the social system of individuals as they move into old age. The first is the role ambiguity associated with moving into the status of "old age"—there is no clearly defined position having associated with it expectancies and taboos. The second is the shrinkage of role repertoires and the decreased activity in roles outside the family."[54] The two roles most often lost are the work role for men and the wife role for women; retirement and widowhood are statuses that indicate a lack of one of life's major roles.

Loss and ambiguity of role may be a step toward the disengagement of the elderly that Elaine Cummings and William Henry, and many others, following them, have discussed. The disengagement theory says that "growing old involves a gradual or inevitable mutual withdrawal or disengagement, resulting in decreased interaction between an aging person and others in the social system he belongs to.

This is double withdrawal—of the individual from society and of the society from the individual."[55] On the other hand, as Arlie Hochschild reports it, the individual "wants" to disengage and does so by reducing the number of roles he plays, lessening the variety of roles, and relationships, and weakening the intensity of those that remain.[56]

Many gerontologists have debated this theory, as Hochschild so aptly reports in her October 1975 article in the American Sociological Review.[57] Studies show wide variations among the aged as to the degree the person withdraws or has lack of interest in activities that subsitute for work. While there is less research on widowhood, most married women become widows, and there is evidence many do not withdraw from society but in fact in a number of cases become more active.

Researchers have found variations in the form as well as the timing of disengagement of the elderly. Sources of variation in disengagement include physiology, personality, type of initial engagement, life situation, and sex role. Moreover, some have found different dimensions of disengagement.[58] For example, Frances Carp found, in studying elderly in a Texas housing complex, that disengagement from family was negatively related to disengagement from social activities and relations with other people.[59] Some found disengagement more related to role loss, widowhood, retirement, and poor health, than to age per se. Hochschild has hypothesized that it is not aging per se that determines disengagement but a combination of factors associated with aging; for example, poor health, widowhood, and other factors associated with the nature of society and one's location in it, which together influence disengagement or engagement.[60]

Disengagement can be replaced by reengagement, such as that of a woman who loses her husband and lifelong friends, but moves into an elderly housing complex and develops a new group of friends. Marion Crawford talks of a group "retiring to something," "released from work and past obligations, enabled to realign with social life outside work and the family," versus a group, more likely working class, who "retire from something" or "retire back to the family."[61]

Not all elderly suffer role loss with retirement; some instead may move to more fulfilling roles as volunteer workers in the work world or as participants in leisure time activities. Some careers, such as teaching, lead one into retirement activities. Furthermore, attitudes toward retirement are becoming more positive in the United States. Eugene Friedman and Harold Orbach report a major shift in outlook toward retirement among U.S. workers in the latter part of the 1950s and throughout the 1960s, with a sharp increase in the proportion of workers reporting favorable attitudes toward retirement. Also, they find the work orientations associated with the job are now shaping concepts of retirement.[62] People are filling time in nonwork activities. Leisure activity is now of more interest and more available to the preretired worker, and this leisure simply increases in the postretirement period. Harold Wilensky sees the work–nonwork relationship in terms of interlocking cycles. Shanas sees nonwork activities as being in terms of time–filling value.[63]

Good social adjustment in terms of changed patterns of behavior —adjusting to new activities, new social roles, and organized life patterns—is becoming more common. Some elderly, due to financial means or flexible psychological orientation, quickly and easily make these changes while others do not.

For the couple that moves into a retirement community, a congregate housing complex, or elderly apartment complex, the lack of occupation and work activities may be easily accepted as all are adapting to this retirement life style.

With knowledge of these adjustment problems due to role loss and ambiguity, the housing complex staff often use various means to encourage reengagement, to stimulate social interaction, and to repromote opportunities for new roles, such as leader of the residents' organization or of a hobby club. Management of a private retirement community may even advertise the complex as having leisure time activities that fill these needs; they may advertise the high status of the residential area. Management of low- and moderate-income elderly housing may try to avoid the buildings getting a negative status, for they know this status will make the elderly more reluctant to become residents.

Even the poorer elderly, concentrated in old housing in certain areas of central cities, may, due to their concentration, not feel challenged to explain their nonwork role. Rosow found that, with increased concentration of the elderly, the working–class elderly, especially those with loss of three or four roles, had a high degree of contact with their neighbors.[64] Role loss did not inhibit contact but led to greater contact.

The poorer elderly may, however, suffer more status loss, due to lower income, possible loss of house, and even loss of automobile. The sudden drop in their financial assets may have a great impact on their self-image. To hold on to a status, keeping up appearances bay be all-important. For some this may mean holding on to a house they can no longer afford to maintain, keeping a car they can no longer drive, or remaining in social clubs they no longer feel part of. Housing allowance assistance, property tax exemptions or .rehabilitation grants or loans, may help them in this effort to hold on to their home.

A final problem some elderly, with serious health and financial limitations, may have is role reversal. Due to senility or physical limitations, these elderly may need to move from their own home to either their children's home or to a congregate living arrangement or nursing home. Often this decision must be made by the adult child. In our Canadian study, only 14 percent of the elderly said relatives helped them decide to move to the complex, but it was felt this was an understatement related to the pride of the elderly;[65] in a nursing home sample, the number receiving help from relatives in making the decision would be much higher.

Not only to the adult children take part in the decision on a move but also many take over financial responsibility and in general guide their parents on decisions. Managers of housing for the elderly must be aware of this reverse role and realize they must contact the adult children on matters affecting their parents.

NOTES

1. Robert Morris, Alternatives to Nursing Home Care: A Proposal, Special Committee on Aging, U.S. Senate, 1st sess., 92d Cong., October 1971; based on data from the 1969 Massachusetts Department of Public Health study.

2. U.S. Department of Commerce, Bureau of the Census, General Population Characteristics, U.S. Summary: 1970 (Washington, D.C.: U.S. Government Printing Office, 1972), Table 49, pp. 1-263; also U.S. Housing Census reported in U.S. Department of Housing and Urban Development, Older Americans: Facts about Income and Housing (Washington, D.C.: U.S. Government Printing Office, October 1963), Tables 2 and 11, p. 26.

3. U.S. Department of Commerce, General Population Characteristics: U.S. Summary 1970, Table 49, pp. 1-263; also U.S. Department of Health, Education and Welfare, Office of Human Development, Administration on Aging, New Facts about Older Americans (Washington, D.C.: U.S. Government Printing Office, June 1973).

4. U.S. Department of Commerce, General Population Characteristics, U.S. Summary 1970, Table 52; U.S. Department of Commerce, Bureau of the Census, Characteristics of the Population, 1960 (Washington, D.C.: U.S. Government Printing Office, 1962), Table 46.

5. Ibid.; also U.S. Department of Housing and Urban Development, Older Americans: Facts about Income and Housing, pp. 32, 34.

6. Business Week, November 20, 1971, p. 57.

7. Barbara Manard, Cary Kart, and Dirk van Gils, Old-Age Institutions (Lexington, Mass.: Lexington Books, 1973), p. 5; also U.S. Department of Commerce, General Population Characteristics, U.S. Summary: 1970, Table 49, pp. 1-263.

8. U.S. Department of Health, Education and Welfare, New Facts about Older Americans; also U.S. Department of Commerce, General Population Characteristics, U.S. Summary: 1970, Table 203.

9. Ibid.

10. Ibid.

11. U.S. Department of Commerce, Bureau of the Census, Detailed Characteristics, U.S. Summary: 1970 (Washington, D.C.: U.S. Government Printing Office, 1972), Table 189.

12. Ibid., Tables 204, 205; also U.S. Department of Housing and Urban Development, Older Americans: Facts about Income and Housing, p. 26.

13. Ethel Shanas, "Living Arrangements and Housing of Old People," in Behavior and Adaptation in Late Life, ed. Ewald Busse and Eric Pfeiffer (Boston: Little, Brown, 1969), pp. 133-35.

14. Michael Audain and Elizabeth Huttman, Beyond Shelter: A Study of NHA-Financed Housing for the Elderly (Ottawa: Canadian Council on Social Development, 1973), pp. 304-06, 334-35.

15. U.S. Department of Commerce, Detailed Characteristics, U.S. Summary: 1970, Tables 245, 259; also U.S. Department of Housing and Urban Development, Older Americans: Facts about Income and Housing; and U.S. Department of Housing and Urban Development, Challenge 6, no. 4 (May 1975), p. 33.

16. Ibid.

17. Shanas, "Living Arrangements and Housing of Old People," p. 140.

18. U.S. Department of Commerce, Bureau of the Census, Subject Report: Housing of Senior Citizens, 1970 (Washington, D.C.: U.S. Government Printing Office, 1972), Tables A-1, A-4.

19. Janet Murray, "Homeownership and Financial Assets: Findings from the 1968 Survey of the Aged," Social Security Bulletin 35, no. 8 (August 1972): 3-23.

20. U.S. Department of Commerce, Bureau of the Census, Housing Characteristics by Household Composition: 1970 (Washington, D.C.: U.S. Government Printing Office, 1973), Tables A-2, B-2, C-2, D-2.

21. U.S. Department of Health, Education and Welfare, Office of Human Development, Administration on Aging, Facts on Aging, Publication 146 (Washington, D.C.: U.S. Government Printing Office, May 1970), p. 20.

22. Ibid., p. 3.

23. Fred Cottrell, Aging and the Aged (Dubuque, Iowa: William C. Brown Co., 1974), p. 8.

24. Margaret Hellie Huyck, Growing Older (Englewood Cliffs, N.J.: Prentice-Hall, 1974), pp. 27-29.

25. Alexander Leaf, "Getting Old," Scientific American 22 (1973): 20.

26. Cottrell, Aging and the Aged, p. 11.

27. Ibid.

28. Jane Brody, "Doctors Study Treatment of Ills Brought on by Stress," New York Times, June 10, 1973, p. 20.

29. Report on the National Health Survey of 1969-70, in U.S. Department of Commerce, Bureau of the Census, The American Almanac: The Statistical Abstract of the United States, 1974 (Washington, D.C.: U.S. Government Printing Office, 1974), Table 125.

30. Audain and Huttman, Beyond Shelter, p. 313.

31. Cope W. Schwenger and L. Allison Sayers, A Sociomedical Study of the Aged, 1965-66 (Toronto: School of Hygiene, University of Toronto, 1969), pp. 60-63, 138.

32. Eric Pfeiffer, "Multi-Dimensional Quantitative Assessment of Three Populations of Elderly" (paper presented at annual meeting of the Gerontological Society, Miami Beach, Fla., November 5-9, 1973).

33. L. Gottesman, M. Moss, and F. Worts, "Resource Needs and Wishes for Services in Urban Middle Class Older People" (paper presented at the Tenth International Congress of Gerontology, Jerusalem, June 22-27, 1975).

34. Ethel Shanas, "Health Status of Older People: Cross-National Implications," American Journal of Public Health 64, no. 3 (March 1974): 261-64.

35. Audain and Huttman, Beyond Shelter, p. 347.

36. Remarks by R. Michael Warren, deputy minister of housing, province of Ontario, reported in "Ontario Regional Workshop on Housing the Elderly; Comments on Housing the Elderly and Beyond Shelter: Proceedings, mimeographed (Ottawa: Canadian Council on Social Development and Ontario Welfare Council, October 1974), p. 9.

37. Marie McGuire Thompson, Design of Housing for the Elderly (Washington, D.C.: National Association of Housing and Urban Redevelopment Officials, 1972), p. 2.

38. U.S. Department of Commerce, Housing Characteristics by Household Composition, 1970, Table A-4.

39. Paul Niebanck, The Elderly in Older Urban Areas (Philadelphia: University of Pennsylvania Press, 1965), p. 42.

40. Richard Sterne, James Phillips, and Alvin Rabushka, The Urban Elderly Poor (Lexington, Mass.: Lexington Books, 1974), p. 23.

41. M. Powell Lawton and Morton Kleban, "The Aged Residents of the Inner City," The Gerontologist 11, no. 4 (1971): 277-84.

42. Irving Rosow, Social Integration of the Aged (New York: The Free Press, 1967), pp. 27, 41.

43. Center for Housing and Environmental Studies, Cornell University, "Community Aspects of Housing for the Aged," mimeographed (Ithaca, N.Y.: Cornell University, 1962).

44. M. Powell Lawton, "Mortality, Morbidity and Voluntary Change of Residence by Older People," Journal of American Geriatric Society 18, no. 10 (October 1970): 823-31; also see David Joyce, Robert Mayer, and Mary Nenno, The Social Functioning of the Dislodged Elderly (Philadelphia: Institute for Environmental Studies, University of Pennsylvania, 1966).

45. Huyck, Growing Older, p. 120.

46. U.S. Department of Commerce, Bureau of the Census, Subject Reports: Housing of Senior Citizens, 1970 (Washington, D.C.: U.S. Government Printing Office, 1974), Tables A-2, B-2, C-2, D-2.

47. Rosow, Social Integration of the Aged, pp. 27, 41.

48. Vern L. Bengtson, The Social Psychology of Aging (Indianapolis: Bobbs-Merrill, 1973), p. 30.

49. R. J. Havighurst, "A Socio-Psychological Perspective of Aging," The Gerontologist 8 (1969).

50. B. L. Neugarten, "Personality Changes in the Aged," Catholic Psychological Record 3 (1965): 13.

51. R. A. Atchley, The Social Forces in Later Life: An Introduction to Social Gerontology (Belmont, Calif.: Wadsworth, 1972), p. 14.

52. Bengtson, The Social Psychology of Aging, p. 29.

53. Ibid., p. 28.

54. Ibid., p. 28; also see Cottrell, Aging and the Aged, pp. 14-15.

55. Elaine Cummings and William Henry, Growing Old (New York: Basic Books, 1961), p. 14.

56. Arlie Hochschild, "Disengagement Theory: A Critique and Proposal," American Sociological Review 40, no. 5 (October 1975): 553-60.

57. Ibid.

58. M. Powell Lawton, Planning and Managing Housing for the Elderly (New York: John Wiley and Sons, 1975), p. 25.

59. Frances Carp, A Future for the Aged: Victoria Plaza and Its Residents (Austin: University of Texas Press, 1966), p. 346.

60. Hochschild, "Disengagement Theory," p. 563.

61. Marion Crawford, "Retirement and Disengagement," Human Relations 24 (1971): 255.

62. Eugene Friedman and Harold Orbach, "Adjustment to Retirement," in The Foundations of Psychiatry, ed. Silvano Arieti (New York: Basic Books, 1974), pp. 614-17.

63. Harold Wilensky, "Life Cycle, Work Situation, and Participation in Formal Associations," in Aging and Leisure, ed. R. W. Kleemeier (New York: Oxford University Press, 1961), pp. 213-42.

64. Rosow, Social Integration of the Aged, pp. 27, 41.

65. Audain and Huttman, Beyond Shelter, p. 321.

CHAPTER

2

NEEDS OF THE ELDERLY

The elderly, like other human beings, have basic common needs such as food, shelter, health care, and opportunities for full growth and interaction with others. As one specialist on the elderly points out, this group's needs can include security—of income, of physical and mental health, and of suitable housing and living arrangements; recognition—as a significant member of society and as an individual with a separately identifiable personality; response and relatedness—the opportunity to relate to others and to be responded to by them; and creativity—to allow fulfillment of the need for exploration and expression of one's capabilities.[1]

Because of the physiological, psychological, and economic limitations given in the preceding chapter, the elderly find some of these needs intensified and above all unmet. For a number there may be a vacuum or inability on their own to adjust and start new roles and develop meaningful activities upon occupational retirement, loss of an independent household, death of a spouse, loss of a position of leadership and status, reduction of income, decrease of physical mobility, loss of living relatives and friends, and possibly movement from a familiar neighborhood. Agencies must step in to meet the needs caused by these changes and losses. Any housing policy for the elderly must take these needs into account, for provision of shelter alone is not enough. For an elderly person to be satisfied with his environment these other needs must be met. We must look beyond shelter.

As the lifespan of the elderly lengthens, we will have in our housing programs an increasing number of persons aged 70 and 80 who will have a wide range of needs stemming from the problems already mentioned. Needs will vary as members of the group will range from those with serious disabilities, causing physical immobility, to

25

healthy older persons with only minor physical frailties. Yet practically all elderly in their seventies and eighties, even if only suffering from minor sorts of infirmities, need help from time to time; the realities of the aging process, as mentioned in Chapter 1, mean that these people develop physiological and psychological deficiencies as time goes on, ranging from frailty and loss of memory to a variety of more serious ailments. Some will suffer such minor handicaps as inability to bend or to climb stairs, while others will develop physical frailties that hinder continuation of heavy housekeeping and maintenance of a large home. For some the home range will contract so that they relate only to their immediate neighborhood, finding the energy expenditure too great for long-distance trips. For some there may also be a disengagement from life, especially withdrawal from social activities.

First, then, previous life style and psychological orientation and, above all, present physical state, much more than chronological age, will determine to what degree the person has these different needs.[2] Second, while the intensity of these needs may increase over time, they may increase due to particular events or crises, such as loss of one's spouse or decrease in financial assets.

To meet these needs a network of services and facilities are required, services that will allow the elderly to maintain their independent living and assure that their welfare is cared for in an atmosphere free of debilitating effects of the institutional world of the nursing home. Services to meet these needs can range from recreational and social animation services to minimal nursing care, to homemaking, and to food preparation. They can range from financial assistance to transportation, to improvement of the neighborhood. The question we deal with in this chapter is which needs are most urgent and should be given the highest priority. Since the list of services could be inexhaustible, while the funding is not, the question as to priorities of need is an important one. The elderly themselves are the best suited to give us these priorities. It is now realized that their values and preferences may differ from those of the professional worker. All too often the practice has been to plan programs for old people without their involvement. We make decisions concerning their life style, ignoring their ability to decide for themselves or express their individual difference. As Rosow has pointed out, "problems of old age are of two general kinds: those that older people actually have and those that experts think they have."[3] In one study postulated on the idea that the elderly themselves will have a different perspective than professionals, it was found in the small sample that services currently offered in Los Angeles County to the elderly did not correspond with the services this group of urban elderly perceived as necessary.[4] In another study with a similar orientation, on the urban poor of Rochester, New York, the researchers came up with similar findings.[5]

The following statement by a council of elderly citizens in the province of Ontario gives some of the reasons why they themselves should be consulted about their priority of needs:

> We the people of Ontario who are over 60 years of age
> number almost one million. . . . We have lived and con-
> tributed for many years to our community and know what
> is important to the quality of life. Now we are experienc-
> ing personally what it means to be elderly. We can see
> areas of great need and identify clearly desirable goals.
> Society tends to deny us the opportunity to participate.
> We insist that greater attention be paid to our views.
> Special services and opportunities are needed to enable
> us to function to the best of our abilities and we believe
> we have the right to participate in their planning so as
> to ensure that these services are designed to meet our
> needs.[6]

The material in this chapter is based on such opinions of the elderly themselves as to need priorities. The bulk of the findings reported come from two separate studies the author has been involved with. These findings are backed up by conclusions from other studies of needs of the elderly, including those of M. B. Hamovitch, J. A. Peterson, and A. E. Larson.[7]

As noted in Chapter 1, the author directed a study that included interviews with 303 elderly in subsidized specially designed apartment complexes and congregate living arrangements across Canada. These elderly were in 19 different developments that were also written up as case studies. In addition, a questionnaire was mailed to a sample of 300 managers of such developments, with 294 responding. A detailed description of this study and its findings has been reported by the author in Beyond Shelter. Besides this four-year nationwide study, the author in 1974 took part in a survey of over 1,200 elderly recipients under the HUD-sponsored experimental housing allowance program (HAP) run by Abt Associates. The data are on elderly in private rented units in eight medium-sized U.S. cities or areas, including two in the South. These surveyed elderly were either participating in the housing allowance experiment or had started application and dropped out; some of them moved from substandard rental units upon entering the program. Thus we have two different groups of elderly, one in private rental units in the community and one sample in specially designed elderly housing.[8]

CHARACTERISTICS OF SURVEYED ELDERLY

In ascertaining the need priorities of the elderly, we must be fully aware of the type of elderly who are giving us these answers. Health status is extremely important, we found, in determining need priorities. In some instances income status may be important, as it may determine whether the elderly person has an unmet need he or she cannot financially afford to meet. However, in this regard it must be kept in mind, first, that in many communities necessary services are often not available even when you have the funds to pay for them. Second, a number of needs are just as urgent and unavailable for the middle-class elderly person as for the poor, with legal and financial assistance being good examples; many well-off widows suffer from lack of accurate information in these areas.

Chronological age is also still a useful criterion for differentiating the elderly, since in a large number of cases there are basic differences between the generation aged 65 to 75 and those over 75, though of a gradual nature and not equally characterizing all members of these age groups. Neugarten, Bengtson, and others[9] have found certain personality and social changes related more to age, compared with other researchers.

Race may also be an important factor influencing need priorities. Richard Sterne, James E. Phillips, and Alvin Rabushka found that two worlds of aging existed side by side in their Model Cities area; that to be old and black was substantially different from being old and white. They found fewer blacks aged 75 and over living in the inner area they studied, because, first, the lower life expectancy of blacks versus whites meant fewer lived to 75, and, second, northern migration of blacks to Rochester was a late phenomenon, so that there were fewer black elderly. These researchers found that white, inner city Rochester elderly had held more satisfactory jobs, owned their own home more often, were better educated, and better off financially than black elderly. Blacks, conversely, were poorer, lived in less satisfactory accommodations, were often dependent on welfare, and were late arrivals.[10] The opinions of black elderly and other minority elderly will be underreported in this book, as they make up a very small percent of the surveyed elderly in both the Canadian study and the HAP study. Most other studies quoted are of white elderly, especially if they are studies of institutionalized elderly, for as Barbara Manard, Cary Kart, and Dirk van Gils point out, blacks are very much underrepresented in institutions for the elderly in the United States. This is due, first, to the fact that there are fewer black elderly, and, second, many of these black elderly are located in the South and rural areas where there are fewer institutions. Lastly, many cannot afford institutions.[11]

The characteristics of the two elderly groups in our studies were that they were a fairly healthy group, with very few in either study having serious health problems, although many of them had some physical limitation; that between a third (the Canadian study) and almost a half (HAP study) said they had trouble getting around; that agewise, in both studies few were under 70 and well over half were over 75. In both cases most of the respondents were not extremely poor, even though they were on housing subsidy programs.

One interesting trait these two groups of elderly had was the lack of many close relatives. In the Canadian group, only a third had spouses living and only half had children living and in the area; for the HAP group, under one-third said they had relatives in the area.

NEED PRIORITIES

In the studies we are focusing on, need priorities were determined in several ways, with similar questions used in both surveys. The elderly were asked what their priorities were, including what they wanted most in any neighborhood they chose to live in; why they were dissatisfied with the neighborhood, housing, and general environment, and why they were satisfied; and, in the Canadian study, why they moved to an elderly housing complex. These elderly were also asked whether they had difficulty doing certain daily tasks, such as housework, cooking, traveling about, and whether they were in need of services (see Table 2.1). Because the focus of these studies was on housing and social services, questions on priorities in these areas were emphasized. The services and facilities required to meet these needs could, in many cases, be given to the person living in his own home and in fact help this person to live an independent life in familiar surroundings, as will be indicated in the chapter on the elderly living in their own home. However, many of these services and facilities also could be utilized by those in specially designed elderly housing complexes, as well be described in the chapters on specially designed elderly apartment complexes and on congregate housing. For some elderly, suffering from the physical limitations mentioned in Chapter 1 and having the needs mentioned in this chapter, specially designed complexes may be the right housing solution, and indeed one that keeps them out of the nursing home. In other words, their limitations, physical, psychological, and social, are severe enough to necessitate a move to the type of shelter where their needs can be more easily met. As James Montgomery states in his article, "The Housing Patterns of Older Families,"

It is an American ideal that older persons should continue to live in their familiar environments for as long as possi-

TABLE 2.1

Health Status, by Development Type

| | Development Type | | |
| | | Self-Contained | |
Health Status	Mixed	Apartments	All
Seriously limited ability[a]			
Number	13	2	15
Percent	7.0	1.7	5.0
Moderately limited ability[b]			
Number	41	12	53
Percent	21.9	10.3	17.5
Slightly limited ability[c]			
Number	70	38	108
Percent	37.4	32.8	35.6
No incapacity[d]			
Number	63	64	127
Percent	33.7	55.2	41.9
Total			
Number	187	116	303
Percent	100	100	100

[a]Seriously limited ability in areas of walking or seeing or hearing; unable to accomplish many daily tasks on own.

[b]Moderately limited physical ability/capacity as noticeable handicap in one activity or faculty mentioned, so person had limited or continuous aid.

[c]Slightly limited physical ability or some minor difficulty either in moving about, communicating, and/or keeping house.

[d]No incapacity (can move about without difficulty) and can keep house.

Note: Interviewer asked resident in depth about his physical limitations and then checked the best-fitting category.

Source: Canadian user survey.

ble. Many aged do cling to the familiar beyond the point in time when reason might dictate a change, and moving may be a major life disruption, socially and psychologically. The limitations of economic resources often militate against repairing and improving dwellings and against

moving to more suitable environments. Generally, programs and services which enable older people to remain
in their present dwellings would be a wise course to follow
for most, but by no means all, aged persons. To make
every effort to enable an impoverished and enfeebled
widow to continue to live in her run-down house or apartment is questionable.[12]

The Need for Income Assistance and/or Cheaper Rents

In discussing priority of needs, one must put the income assistance need at the top of the list for many elderly. One must also realize it is a need that directly and indirectly influences the person's
ability to utilize many need-meeting services, including the abovementioned maintenance of his or her home. As Ontario elderly state:
"We need enough money to pay our rent . . . we need to be able to
buy proper food to keep healthy, and to meet medical expenses and
drug costs. We should be able to buy presentable clothing, to pay for
transportation, and have something left over for emergencies, plea-
sures. . . . The actual amount required will depend upon free or reduced cost of services made available."[13]
The income limitations of the elderly in our population has already been mentioned in Chapter 1. Therefore it is not surprising to
find it a top priority need of surveyed elderly. Of major importance
to the surveyed U.S. elderly who take part, to varying degrees, in
the HUD-sponsored housing allowance experiment, was the need for
assistance in meeting their rent bill. When asked about their great
need in locating housing, the largest group mentioned finding a place
they could afford. For a number a problem with their present house
was that the "rent was too high"; a fifth mentioned this. Those who
had previously owned housing said the reason for selling was that it
was too expensive; over half the previous owners mentioned this.
Most who wanted to move out of their present housing said the reason
for selling was that it was too expensive; over half the previous owners
mentioned this. Most who wanted to move out of their present housing
said the main reason they did not move was that they could not find an
apartment at the rent they could afford. Many had a very high rent-
income burden. They also found the costs of moving to a new unit,
as well as the expense of the security deposit for the unit, a serious
problem.
The Canadian elderly also expressed concern over money. These
elderly gave as their major reason for coming to the subsidized housing developments the fact that they felt "it was financially the best
housing choice" in view of their limited income or simply that it was

"cheap rent." They also gave this as a reason for satisfaction with the house.

In a small survey (mentioned above) of urban elderly poor in Rochester, the researchers' conclusion was that "the potentially most rewarding way to assist many of the elderly poor was to give them increased cash, a desire expressed by many old people during our community interviews."[14]

Need for Accessibility to Services or Transportation to Services

While "problem with transportation" was not the most serious problem with this Rochester sample, it was one that almost a fourth of the 75-year-olds and over mentioned and in fact a fourth of the black elderly mentioned. In other studies, including our own, this and accessibility to services have turned out to be very high priority needs among the range of needs of the surveyed elderly.

Accessibility to services often becomes a main concern when energy resources of the person decline so that lengthy freeway or bus trips are hard to make. Immobility, which occurs when the person develops physical handicaps that make it hard for him to board a bus or operate a car or take long taxi rides, may heighten interest in accessibility.

Concern with accessibility to services was expressed in a variety of ways by the elderly in our two studies. The Canadian elderly gave, as an important reason for satisfaction or dissatisfaction with their specially designed elderly housing, the accessibility of the house to services. A third of this group felt their housing was so located as not to make easy access to important services. On another question, a sizable group said they were not satisfied with location, with their main reason being that it was "far from stores." A major reason, on the other hand, for being satisfied with the development was that it was in a "convenient location." The researchers interviewing these elderly in each case assessed the development's suitability for each person; these interviewers felt some developments were unsuitable because they were not close to shopping and residents needed transportation services. The inaccessibility of outer area housing developments to services seemed to closely correlate with the degree to which elderly in such developments got out daily. Those in inner area developments were much more likely to get out one hour or more daily and to participate in some community activities; they were also more satisfied with their housing (see Chapter 8 for an expansion of this discussion). The HAP surveyed elderly gave accessibility to services as the major criterion for a satisfactory neighborhood and gave types of services they wanted nearby.

This question is of course a basic one. What types of services do the elderly most often want accessible to them? In the Hamovitch, Peterson, and Larson study, over 90 percent of the total large sample (718 elderly in four types of housing) considered the location of their housing in relation to community facilities, such as shopping and other services, to be very important or somewhat important.[15] Both our samples were most concerned that shopping services be accessible. For example, when asked what special feature they looked for and needed in locating any place to live, well over half of the HAP elderly said convenience to shopping.

The next priority as to what service should be close, mentioned by a smaller group, was "a place close to a doctor, clinic, or hospital." In the Canadian study these elderly were again especially concerned with accessibility to health services. The Rochester elderly poor surveyed by Sterne, Phillips, and Rabushka were also found to have as the second most often mentioned concern "trouble seeing a doctor," possibly indicating an accessibility problem. In addition, one of this group's great mobility problems was expressed in terms of it being "hard to go shopping." Almost a third, aged 65–74, said shopping was hard to do, as did 39 percent of those 75 and over.[16] In our samples difficulties also increased with age, although they were even more closely related to health status. In the Hamovitch, Peterson, and Larson study, the proportion of the group considering it important to be located close to professional persons or services varied by income status, with only two-thirds of the welfare group considering it important, compared to 86 percent of the retirement community group.[17]

Accessibility to a place of worship or a library or a park or a senior center was far less important to our two groups of elderly. In fact, in the HAP survey few, when questioned, were worried about whether the neighborhood they moved to had a senior center, a place of worship, or other recreational places.

Accessibility to relatives and friends, surprisingly, was not a major concern to either group. In the Canadian study only 40 percent of those with children considered whether they lived in the same neighborhood as their children "very important"; a large proportion, 44 percent, had no living children or none living in the area. The Hamovitch, Peterson, and Larson study came up with similar findings. First, a surprisingly large proportion had no children, and, second, a relatively small percentage of those with children thought it important for their housing to be located near their children, and they were even less concerned about living near other relatives.[18]

Accessibility could relate to degree of interaction with relatives. In our Canadian study, even though many of the specially designed developments were not located near where relatives lived (though they were more likely to be if they were downtown developments or rural developments), still there was a high degree of interaction with relatives. Yet in the survey of Rochester urban poor, the researchers found a main concern to be the "problems of visiting families," with a fifth of those under 75 mentioning it and almost a third of those 75 and over.[19]

Transportation is of course important if the elderly person is located in an inaccessible area, such as an outer fringe or a suburban area of the city, or in a rural community. A very large proportion of the elderly, especially those over 75, do not own or drive an automobile; the proportion ranges from almost half in one national study to three-fourths in our study of congregate elderly. Thus, lack of public transportation can be a barrier to free movement for many elderly, locking them into restricted environments. On the other hand, if good transportation services exist, this can increase mobility and make services needed more accessible. The elderly in our samples considered good transportation services a high priority need. In the HAP study they gave this need a top ranking and gave as the most important feature of any neighborhood its nearness to good transportation services, as well as to grocery stores. In both studies many had difficulty getting places (a third to a half) and this caused a concern over transportation. In the HAP study, of those who moved into a new neighborhood after receiving a housing allowance, their biggest problem was finding transportation to required services, followed by a related problem, that of seeing relatives. These HAP participants also said one of their biggest problems in trying to utilize the program was getting someone to drive them around to look at housing; they wanted also to be counseled as to what apartments were near transportation routes.

In the Canadian study a number felt a need for a better bus system, especially if they were in outer or suburban areas. They complained the bus stops were too far away or there were limited stops, infrequent service, or poor routing. A reason they gave for dissatisfaction with the elderly housing was need for transportation service. Only 15 percent said a voluntary transportation service was available, and this was mainly to church and often available only to a few special persons. In some cases they used a taxi as a group or had relatives and friends drive them to needed services. The few cases where outer area developments or a related agency supplied transportation, as with one Montreal development, were cases where the rate of getting out daily one hour or more was higher than for other outer area developments.

Both the needs for accessible services and transportation were less likely to be mentioned by the group of elderly that said they did not get out or they had difficulty getting around. For the nonambulatory elderly the services must come to them rather than having them go to the services. In Chapter 8 we will expand on this. For the individual handicapped person some special van or other transportation that comes upon call or by appointment might be of use.

Health Needs

Health needs are of major concern to the elderly, who continually fear that their mobility will be sharply decreased by a sickness or that medical aid will not be readily available in an emergency situation. They also fear the costs of the hospitalization will be such to wipe out their savings, even though they are covered by Medicare. In 1969 the medical bills of the U.S. elderly came to almost $14 billion and only 70 percent of that was covered by Medicare, Medicaid, or any private health plan.[20] It is no wonder U.S. elderly consider coverage of all medical costs a major need.

In our studies, especially the Canadian one, the need was expressed in terms of wanting someone available in times of health emergencies and, in a number of cases, having a nurse visit once a week. The Canadian elderly feared they might become sick with no one knowing of their illness. They gave examples of persons who had become ill and gone for hours without help. One case mentioned by elderly in a Toronto development was that of

> an older lady who fell in her apartment on Sunday morning and had broken her arm. She became unconscious. There was no staff on Sunday and none of us visited her. It wasn't till afternoon that she was conscious enough to call out and for us to finally hear her. Since there was no staff on Sunday, we didn't know where to call. We finally got a doctor through the hospital.

Many of the residents of this development repeated this same story to our interviewers. It indicated they had a desire for the security of a setting where staff were available to help. In the Canadian survey many, when asked, said they expected to turn to development staff when an emergency arose; a large number had no relatives to turn to. About a fifth of this group said they needed nursing staff on a regular basis. The need was less likely if they were in apartments and was greater in congregate housing serving those with more health problems; it was less likely if children were in the area or if a spouse was living with the person. For a number, the need was not immediate health assistance but just the availability of it for future needs. Some said they would like a room with a buzzer that connected with the man-

ager's office; a large group would prefer a housing complex that included a nursing wing, presumably so they could move to it when they
became sick. This particular preference was also given by the majority of the HAP elderly.

Other indications that health needs were of major concern to
the Canadian elderly were that some said they came to the development because of these needs; some said they were satisfied with the
development because it offered some medical help, as congregate
housing usually did. As already mentioned, both groups gave high
priority to having the medical offices near them.

In other reports, elderly have given, as part of their health
needs, the need for medical and dental insurance that covers all costs,
the need for medical screening examinations, and the need for health
education, counseling, and referral. They would like community
health clinics that would cater to their needs; many feel doctors often
give them little attention and even are unwilling to serve them, especially if they are under Medicaid, and they think the existence of a
special clinic could improve this situation.[21]

Needs Centering Around Difficulty with
Housing, Cooking, and Shopping

Slower movements, memory loss, and physical limitations
make it hard for some elderly to push a vacuum cleaner, cook a large
meal, or do the supermarket shopping and carry the grocery bags
home. In our Canadian elderly sample, almost a fourth admitted difficulty with cooking, almost a third difficulty with housework, and an
equal proportion difficulty in shopping in winter. These are high
proportions for a group that is ambulatory. This degree of need is
verified by the fact that 16 percent of these elderly said they actually
came to the development because they needed assistance in these
areas. Those who moved into congregate arrangements were more
likely to have this need, and of course had the need met in such a development, with its dining room and maid service. However, almost
a fifth of the apartment dwellers had difficulty doing housework, and
a few had a service available to meet this need. Few of the apartment
dwellers who had difficulty cooking used a meals-on-wheels service;
those who had difficulty shopping did, in a number of cases, use a
grocery delivery service. In another studied sample, that of Rochester urban poor, difficulty with shopping was also a major problem
for about 40 percent of the 75 and over age group.[22]

Need for Social Interaction

Retirement from a job and/or loss of a spouse may cause a
considerable drop in social interaction for the elderly person. He or

she may have trouble initiating new contacts and developing new friendships. The person withdraws from active participation in the community; he or she does not turn to leisure activities to replace former workplace activities. Then reduction in social contacts may cause the person to voluntarily resign from life and even stop caring for basic needs, such as provision of his or her own meals, cleaning the house, or proper attention to medical needs. The person may realize this need, saying he or she feels lonely or isolated. Over a fifth of our surveyed Canadian elderly said they came to the development because "they needed company, felt depressed, lonely or isolated" or "wanted to be close to other people in the development." Half of the single residents in the development had lived with a spouse before coming to the development. Almost a half had no children or none living in the area. When in the development, many gave as their reason for satisfaction with it the fact that it was a "friendly atmosphere" and a place in which it was "easy to make friends."

Elderly in their own home also have this need for social interaction. Social service organizations try in various ways to reach out to them; for example, Bellevue Hospital in New York City has a program in a center on the Lower East Side to reach out to the frail and isolated elderly in that area.

Other programs focus on younger active elderly, seeing their need in terms of recreational leisure time activities to fill the gap left, timewise, by retirement, and at the same time to provide both mental and physical stimulation. One of the ten major needs given by a group of active elderly representatives on an Ontario council was

the need for multi-purpose senior citizen centers with their use to include "providing for a full range of social, educational and cultural needs" and "opportunity for meaningful use of leisure time" as well as "the greatest opportunity for participation in planning and for the delivery of services.[23]

Need for Interaction in the Neighborhood and for a Desirable Neighborhood

From the perspective of the aging adult the neighborhood is his world. His home range has contracted and he increasingly uses only local shops and services. This environment can give him a feeling of pleasure and a feeling of place or can be stressful with its noise, dirt, and strangers.

As age increases, the person may depend more on local friendships; so he wants neighbors of his own age and type, as the majority in both our studies did. Rosow[24] points out that, with advanced age, there is an increasing dependence on local neighborhood friendship ties, and people are most satisfied when they have such ties and when there is a high concentration of elderly in the neighborhood. In our HAP study elderly who did have friends living nearby, and the majority of this group did, were much more likely to be very satisfied with the neighborhood than those who did not have friends nearby. Fewer of these elderly had relatives living nearby, and the presence or absence of relatives seemed to have little effect on their satisfaction with the neighborhood. The elderly in this study, and in the Hamovitch-Peterson-Larson study, when asked, did not seem to consider it necessary to have relatives and, in fact, friends living near them, showing a contradictory situation.

Satisfaction with physical aspects of the neighborhood is also a need, but what is a "desirable" or "satisfactory" neighborhood may not always be based on the criteria the planner would normally take into account. While a pleasing green area, with standard housing, may appeal to many elderly, in some cases it might be outweighed by the fact that the neighborhood is familiar—has the same shops the elderly person has patronized for years, the same park and even park bench, the same long-term residents.

Certainly for the elderly who are willing to move or psychologically flexible enough to move, green lawns, parklike atmosphere, and a comfortable modern housing complex are important. Our Canadian elderly who had moved to outer area developments with such features were pleased with the location. HAP movers also appreciated the better area. In the Hamovitch-Peterson-Larson study, the subsample living in a middle-class retirement community, 100 miles from Los Angeles, only ten years old, and with a variety of recreation facilities, were considerably more satisfied with location, including terrain and view, than the subsamples of welfare recipients, either dispersed in an inner city area or in a downtown residential hotel, as well as a sample of dispersed retired moderate-income employees. Over three-fourths of all of the Hamovitch-Peterson-Larson groups thought location was very or somewhat important.[25] Yet it was those willing to move and with the financial means to move that found a satisfactory environment, in terms of landscaping, recreational facilities, and nondeteriorated housing. Many elderly Americans make the move every year to such elderly complexes as Leisure World, or to resort areas, such as St. Petersburg, Florida, especially to get such an environment as well as a warm climate.

Yet for many elderly a satisfactory location and neighborhood is one that is familiar even if it is deteriorating. The rate of residential mobility among elderly is very low and much lower than that for the whole U.S. population. A Social Security Administration survey showed 80 percent of the couples over the age of 62 had lived for more than ten years in their present community.[26] Study after study show the elderly have had long-term residence in the same house. Elderly in owner-occupied units are more likely to be long-term residents than those in rental units; in 1970, nearly half the households with elderly heads, if owner-occupiers, had been in the same house 20 years.[27] Many elderly want to stay in the same neighborhood, even if it is a badly deteriorating one, as certainly is the case for many inner city and rural areas that elderly inhabit; the elderly give these areas high ratings as satisfactory neighborhoods as found in study after study. Lawton and Kleban gave several reasons why the elderly seem to have been so satisfied with the Philadelphia low-income, extremely deteriorated neighborhood surveyed: preference for familiar surroundings; memory of life as it used to be in the area; high degree of homeownership and strong attachment to home; existence of a large peer group. Lawton and Kleban found that, of the aged who do change residences, most remained in the same neighborhood.[28] A sense of place, as Montgomery points out, is a basic need of many elderly.[29] They, more than other groups, have the need for the sense of spatial identity Marc Fried speaks of,[30] the sense of relatedness to a group, and sense of mastery of the physical environment, found in a familiar setting.[31] These factors may explain why most in our HAP sample were satisfied with their present neighborhood (we did find that those who had moved to different housing when getting the allowance were slightly more likely to be satisfied). Since many of these elderly lived in inner city areas, it was surprising not only that three-fourths felt it was a very satisfactory neighborhood but that well over three-fourths said that there was a low crime level in the area, good police protection, well-kept streets and sidewalks, low level of noise, and, even in greater number, that most houses and yards were well kept and neat. Of course some elderly seldom leave their home and thus view the neighborhood from this perspective. Moreover, some of these elderly are living in older inner areas but ones that are modestly kept up, especially in the smaller surveyed cities such as Salem, Oregon, and Bismarck, North Dakota.

Dissatisfaction does of course exist among some inner city elderly. Some are bothered because redevelopment has occurred and they are moved to other areas than those they are not familiar with. Our HAP group of movers worried about the transportation and shopping facilities in their new areas. Sterne's white elderly, while not moving, were in some cases worried about the change of racial composition in the area. He reports that about an equal proportion of blacks and whites (about one-third) expressed displeasure with these inner city Rochester neighborhoods, but, he adds, as the racial composition of the neighborhood became increasingly black, white displeasure dramatically rose:

> Whites living on blocks with few or no blacks are happy
> with their neighborhood. Those unhappy more than dou-
> ble as the neighborhood takes on an evenly mixed racial
> tone. Finally, three out of four whites are unhappy liv-
> ing in what are virtually black or Puerto Rican neighbor-
> hoods, a rate of unhappiness about fivefold greater than
> for whites living in white majority areas.[32]

He adds that "a similar analysis for blacks does not disclose a strong
relationship between residential propinquity to whites and happiness
with the neighborhood." Sterne points out that whites who were unhappy wanted to move "while for blacks, unhappiness with the neighborhood was expressed not in terms of escape from the area, but in the
desire to see improvement in the physical character of the area and
greater personal security."

The increased incidence of crime and concern over safety are
indeed points of interest to inner city elderly. Many no longer go out
at night due to the criminal activities in their area. Some have their
Social Security checks stolen or their homes broken into. Sterne
says "purse-snatching, house break-ins, the quest for personal security describe precisely the world of the urban elderly poor."[33]
This situation causes the elderly person to be in constant fear. Joel
D. Aberbach and Jack Walker report on one resident's statement on
a Detroit inner city area:

> The neighborhood had changed profoundly during the forty
> years she had lived there. It had once been full of families
> she knew and trusted but now was inhabited by strangers;
> it had been all white and now was almost all black. She
> found this change in her environment deeply threatening;
> hers was a life of almost perpetual fear. She reported
> that during the year before our interview her purse had
> been stolen from her twice on the street and her house
> had been broken into once. . . . Her declining energies
> and prospects, her poverty, her unhappiness at changes
> taking place all around her, led to a powerful yearning for
> personal security. Policemen "should walk their beats.
> We need more police protection, instead of just driving by
> real fast." . . . When asked about the best possible life
> imaginable she said: "I would just like to live free of fear.
> I want to know I can walk the streets and be safe either day
> or night. I don't want to be scared every time the bell
> rings."[34]

Similar worries about security have been expressed by elderly public
housing tenants. For example, in a public housing project for the el-

derly in the San Francisco Tenderloin district, a skid row-deviant behavior area, so many unpleasant incidents occurred to the elderly
tenants of the modest project that they demanded 24-hour security
guards and elaborate lock systems. In a number of projects elderly
are mixed with families and the teenage youth cause problems. In a
White Plains, New York, project where the elderly had one whole
floor, they feared to leave that floor and especially to use the elevator.
    If neighborhood is such an important focus for the elderly's
world, these various needs related to it should be met. It should be
clean with decent lighting, parks, familiar buildings, possibly a concentration of elderly, and it should be a safe place to live.
    In summarizing this chapter, we must point out that basic needs
must be met if the housing environment is to be a satisfactory one for
the elderly person. While shelter is certainly a major need, and one
we focus on in the next chapter, other important needs stand alongside
it.

NOTES

    1. Donald P. Kent, "Social Services and Social Policy," in
Aging and Social Policy, ed. John C. McKinney and Frank T. deVyver
(New York: Appleton-Century-Crofts, 1966), pp. 208-11.
    2. B. L. Neugarten, "Personality and Patterns of Aging," in
Neugarten, Middle Age and Aging (Chicago: University of Chicago
Press), pp. 173-77; Vern Bengtson, The Social Psychology of Aging
(Indianapolis: Bobbs-Merrill, 1973), p. 33.
    3. Irving Rosow, Social Integration of the Aged (New York:
The Free Press, 1967), p. 2.
    4. Mark Riesenfeld et al., "Perceptions of Public Service
Needs: The Urban Elderly and the Public Agency," The Gerontologist
12 (Summer 1972): pt. 1, 185-90.
    5. Richard Sterne, James E. Phillips, and Alvin Rabushka,
The Urban Elderly Poor (Lexington, Mass.: D. C. Heath, 1973),
pp. 80-81, 86-88.
    6. "The Elderly Define Their Goals," Ontario Welfare Reporter
19 (Spring 1973): 4-5.
    7. M. B. Hamovitch, J. A. Peterson, and A. E. Larson,
"Perceptions and Fulfillment of Housing Needs of an Aging Population"
(paper presented at Eighth International Congress of Gerontology,
Washington, D.C., August 26, 1969).
    8. Michael Audain and Elizabeth Huttman, Beyond Shelter: A
Study of NHA-Financed Housing for the Elderly (Ottawa: Canadian
Council on Social Development, 1973). This was a report of a nation-
wide study of specially designed subsidized apartments and congregate

housing for the elderly. The special survey of elderly participating
in the HUD-sponsored housing allowance experiment was done in
Salem, Oregon; Bismarck, North Dakota; Durham, North Carolina;
Springfield, Massachusetts; Jacksonville, Florida; Tulsa, Oklahoma;
Peoria, Illinois; and San Bernardino County, California. The number
surveyed varied by question as not all respondents were asked all
questions but the overall number was over 1,200, 965 of them actually
becoming recipients and the rest applicants. The author was consultant to the project and designed a number of questions and helped anal-
yze the data in the summer of 1974.

9. Neugarten, "Personality and Patterns of Aging," pp. 173-77
Bengtson, The Social Psychology of Aging, p. 34.

10. Sterne, Phillips, and Rabushka, The Urban Elderly Poor,
p. 84.

11. Barbara Manard, Cary Kart, and Dirk van Gils, Old-Age
Institutions (Lexington, Mass.: D. C. Heath, 1974), p. 44.

12. James Montgomery, "The Housing Patterns of Older Families," The Family Coordinator 21 (January 1972): 41.

13. "The Elderly Define Their Goals," p. 4.

14. Sterne, Phillips, and Rabushka, The Urban Elderly Poor,
pp. 27, 87.

15. Hamovitch, Peterson, and Larson, "Perceptions and Fulfillment of Housing Needs," p. 8.

16. Sterne, Phillips, and Rabushka, The Urban Elderly Poor,
pp. 27, 57.

17. Hamovitch, Peterson, and Larson, "Perceptions and Fulfillment of Housing Needs," p. 10.

18. Ibid.

19. Sterne, Phillips, and Rabushka, The Urban Elderly Poor,
p. 27.

20. "Special Report on Old People," Business Week, November
20, 1971, pp. 56-57.

21. "The Elderly Define Their Goals," p. 4.

22. Sterne, Phillips, and Rabushka, The Urban Elderly Poor,
p. 27.

23. "The Elderly Define Their Goals," p. 4.

24. Rosow, Social Integration of the Aged, pp. 27-41.

25. Hamovitch, Peterson, and Larson, "Perceptions and Fulfillment of Housing Needs," p. 7.

26. Calvin Goldscheider, "Differential Residential Mobility of
the Older Population," Journal of Gerontology 21 (January 1966): 103-
08.

27. Manard, Kart, and van Gils, Old-Age Institutions, p. 23.

28. M. Powell Lawton and Morton Kleban, "The Aged Resident
of the Inner City," The Gerontologist 11 (1971): 277-84.

29. Montgomery, "The Housing Patterns of Older Families,"
p. 40.

30. Marc Fried, "Grieving for a Lost Home," in The Urban
Condition, ed. Leonard Duhl (New York: Basic Books, 1963), pp.
151-71.

31. Montgomery, "The Housing Patterns of Older Families,"
pp. 39-41.

32. Sterne, Phillips, and Rabushka, The Urban Elderly Poor,
pp. 35-36.

33. Ibid., p. 69.

34. Joel D. Aberbach and Jack Walker, Race in the City (Boston: Little, Brown, 1972), pp. 98-99.

CHAPTER
3

HOUSING CONDITIONS
AND HOUSING NEEDS
OF THE ELDERLY

A major need of the elderly in the United States is comfortable, reasonable housing designed and located to compensate for some of their physical, psychological, and economic limitations. Their needs range from the psychological ones of safety and comfort, a sense of place, relatedness, and environmental mastery,[1] to those related to physical limitations, such as design features like elevators, ramps, an adequate heating system, and easy maintenance units, to social concerns such as homogeneous grouping, landlord relations, tenant contacts and privacy, and safety from strangers.

A basic need is a sense of place, that is, to feel the unit is your unit, one that you can identify with. It should be a place that either is a familiar surrounding or quickly becomes familiar, with the elderly person able to relate to the people living there and to the environment. The need is for independence that allows the elderly to be master of their own household. In most cases this need should be met by keeping the elderly in their own home. In some cases, because of the aged's physical and mental condition, other housing alternatives are more suitable, but in such cases the person should be given a sense of place in his new home. The elderly need environmental mastery in whatever unit they are in.[2] This may mean ability to furnish it as they wish, decorate the unit, or put in whatever garden they want. Unfortunately the nursing home and some congregate living arrangements do not allow this.

Another need of the elderly is to have housing they take pride in. A number are willing to move from their familiar unit in a slum area to a new apartment complex or retirement home to get this. Because of this need for a home they can be proud of, they may not be interested in public housing or even Section 236 housing because of the stigma these programs have. In the HAP study, less than 10 percent

said, when asked if they had a choice, would they "rather live in public housing or private housing," that they would be interested in public housing, even though this was a low-income eligible group.

A basic need the elderly have is for a choice of housing alternatives. A number of writers[3] have pointed out the need to provide
housing consistent with a variety of life styles and with a variety of
physical or health levels. This choice variable is discussed at length
in the next chapter, on types of housing now being planned for the elderly and types of subsidy programs. Most experts agree the choice
is too limited today.[4]

HOUSING DESIGN

The declining functional capacity of the elderly means that safety
and health features must be built into their home environment. Home
accidents are a major cause of illness and even death in our society,
with over 17 million people needing medical care for home accidents
each year. The elderly, with their reduced sensory ability and with
their serious mobility problems, are especially liable to have accidents and in many cases they have more severe injuries causing hospitalization, or a long period with a cast or cane; such accidents may
end the elderly's ability to stay in their own home. Because of their
vulnerability to falls and other accidents their units should be equipped
to minimize injury. One report has categorized their health problems
in terms of mobility-agility, touch sensation, sight problems, hearing problems, and smell sensation.[5] It points out that the elderly
need to conserve energy, in terms of lifting, bending, pulling, or climbing; need to be safe from hazardous housing conditions; need to have
an adequate temperature-climate control; need to be protected from
bothersome level of noise; and need to be provided with adequate space
for various activities. It also suggests the need for security.[6] These
needs relate to a lessened ability to climb stairs or handle curbs, to
reach high cupboards, to carry heavy loads or lift objects, to see or
to read small print, and to hear, including hearing telephones, alarms,
and doorbells. The fact their mobility is limited and their hearing often deteriorated means that there is also a need for fire safety measures. The fact that the elderly have low resistance to respiratory
ailments means heat must be controlled. The fact that many have a
decreased sense of balance and occasional dizziness means they need
wall supports and resting places.[7] The fact that the elderly are more
susceptible to arthritis, rheumatism, high blood pressure, diabetes,
and heart disease means the need for easy accessibility to the unit.
The fact that they have serious diseases and frequent accidents that
lead to long periods of confinement or limited mobility means their

housing unit is the major center of their lives and needs to be pleasant and comfortable. Space should be appealing in terms of size,
shape, color, and outlook or view: it should be designed for those
with wheelchairs or walking aids and for those with poor eyesight
and/or hearing problems. Design features to meet all these needs
will be discussed in Chapter 7.

One need mentioned in many studies is an elevator or one-floor
unit. In both our studies most of the elderly gave this as a definite
need, with 96 percent of the HAP group saying they wanted all rooms
on one floor. Another need expressed in the HAP study was heat,
with a number feeling they lacked adequate heating in the winter.

For some the need might be for housing with a communal dining
facility, and for others, housing that had a nursing wing or nearby
nursing or medical facility. In the HAP study of elderly private renters, over a third said they would like housing with communal dining
facilities. In our Canadian study many in congregate housing of course
had such facilities but a number in the apartment units would like
them. In both studies there was an indication the residents would
like medical care either nearby or in another wing of the building. In
the Canadian study 72 percent favored a multicare housing complex
that included a nursing wing; those with seriously limited physical
ability, in 89 percent of the cases, "definitely favor" such a complex,
while only 33 percent of those with no physical incapacity "definitely
favor" it, although another 39 percent of this group "somewhat favor" it. The dining and medical facility issues will be discussed in a
later chapter.

The elderly also had a need for privacy. In the Canadian study,
among the few not happy with the degree of privacy the real problem
was sharing a room or a bathroom. Those who shared were quite
dissatisfied with it. Due to their health problems they disliked sharing a bathroom. Most were happy with the degree of privacy, mentioning it as a reason for satisfaction with the development, and, in
mentioning it, indicating this variable was an important one to them.

A related need was that of having a homogeneous group in the
building, and not families with young children. In the HAP study
about a third of the private elderly renters preferred age-segregated
housing, while in the Canadian study of elderly who had already moved
into age-segregated buildings, 89 percent said they would prefer to
live in a building with their own age group. Thus this need varies
from sample to sample, as discussed in a later chapter.

There may also be a need to have areas for interaction such as
a mailbox area, an inviting lobby or a comfortable, livable lounge,
as well as a laundry room. There may be a need for areas that the
elderly can call their own such as garden plots, floor kitchens, lounge
nooks on each corridor of each floor, or, in warm climates, balconies.

A major need is for easy maintenance units. As already indicated, health problems make it difficult for the elderly to maintain
large old homes. Above all other reasons, the Canadian elderly said
they came to the developments because they had had maintenance
problems in their past housing (and because they needed a cheaper
unit, a fact that can be related to maintenance costs). The HAP elderly who had owned a house in the past said a major reason for selling it was the maintenance problems.

A number of elderly would take a smaller unit to get away from
these maintenance problems. Few elderly in either study found moving to a smaller unit a factor that bothered them. However, there
are differences in opinions, as mentioned in the chapter on specially
designed apartments, as to the acceptability of studio units.[8] While
many elderly accept the fact that a small accommodation may be more
convenient and efficient, and be at a rent they can afford, they feel a
studio apartment is too compact and they need a one-bedroom unit;
other elderly accept the studio.

A desire or need these elderly very definitely have is for a
comfortable modern unit that is easy to maintain and is pleasant and
livable. The newness of the unit very much appeals to elderly who
have lived in old deteriorating housing. A large proportion of our
Canadian elderly said a major reason they moved to the housing development was that it was a "comfortable modern home" (see Table
3.1). In the HAP sample many of those who had moved were now in
higher-standard housing than before the move; this group was more
satisfied with their housing than those who had not moved.

A last need is to find this comfortable modern unit, with the
design features mentioned, at a rent the elderly can afford. Since
over half of elderly headed renter households in the United States in
1970 had a gross income of less than $3,000,[9] this meant they could
only pay, at the most, $750 a year for rent if they paid 25 percent of
their income for rent; many elderly of course have even less than
$3,000 gross income a year and thus even this $750, or $63 a month,
rent comes to more than a fourth of their income. At any rate the
question is, Where can this half of the elderly population find a comfortable modern unit for $63 a month? The next section describes the
kind of housing they actually get and what proportion of their income
they use for it.

HOUSING CONDITIONS OF THE ELDERLY

In contrast to housing needs of the elderly, we have the present
condition of the housing that the elderly in the United States now live
in. This is a startling contrast. Only a very small proportion of the

TABLE 3.1

Reasons for Moving to Development

Reason	Number Giving Reason*
Felt financially it was best housing choice (including reasonable rent)	105
Unable to keep up maintenance of own home (previous house too roomy)	82
Security and safety	67
Needed help in cooking, shopping, home-making	48
Wanted more comfortable or modern housing than former accommodation	48
Needed company (formerly lonely, depressed, or isolated)	43
Relatives, social agency, doctor, friends/ neighbors, encourged entry	40
Needed nursing/medical services	32
Planned move as part of retirement	31
Previously living with family who needed room, or made them feel uncomfortable (19 cases), or housing rules made move necessary when spouse died	28
Preferred location (for example, close to children, relatives, or downtown)	25
Loss of previous home (due to expropriation or financial need to sell)	25
Wanted to be close to other people in development	23
Too many steps in previous accommodation	12

*Some residents gave more than one response.

Source: Canadian user survey.

elderly live in specially designed housing of any type. A half million subsidized elderly units of one type or another had been built by 1975; 273,270 of these in 1975 were specially designed elderly housing units, and another equally large group consisted of convenient units in mixed housing occupied by elderly public housing tenants. Another large group was Section 202, 202/236 or 236. In 1973 the National Center for Housing Management reported that 44,500 units were Section 202

housing, 28,500 were 202/236 housing, and the rest, 236 housing of
a total of over 400 million subsidized units.[10] About 5 percent of our
elderly population, or a million people, live in group quarters—nursing homes and homes for the aged or other facilities—with most of these
in nursing homes. A 1974 estimate was that there were only 400 congregate living complexes in all of the United States.[11] This is in contrast to the 120,000 units of new elderly housing a year recommended
by the White House Conference on Aging in 1971 in its Housing the
Elderly report.

Is there serious need for this new housing? All statistics indicate there is. But first let us look at the living arrangements and
tenure at present for most elderly households. Most elderly live in
housing units (95 percent), not group quarters, and almost 70 percent
own their own home. Less than 30 percent rent their unit.[12]

Regarding living arrangements, while 70.8 percent of all elderly live in family units where they either are related to the household hear or are the head themselves, a fair number of these are living in the home of a relative rather than their own home; almost two
million live with adult children.[13] For those widowed who have living
children, almost a half of them live with these children. We know
from studies that this is not always a desirable situation for either the
elderly parent or the adult children who have their own family to care
for. The situation can cause conflict or reversal of the parent-child
role where the adult child who owns the home now becomes the com-
manding figure. In a number of cases the elderly parent has health
problems, including senility and immobility, that present serious care
problems to the adult child. With the increase in day care centers,
we are finding a number of these families resorting to such help.[14]

While 13.5 million elderly in 1970 lived in these family households where the elderly person or a relative was head, this still
leaves over 6.5 million U.S. elderly living in some other arrangement. Of these the largest group are living alone or with unrelated
individuals, such as boarders in independent households; over 5.5
million were in this category in 1970.[15] That a fourth of the elderly
population is living alone (or in some cases with boarders or unrelated persons) has a variety of consequences. We already discussed
how a number have difficulty cooking, cleaning, and maintaining their
home, and have health problems; it is easy to project from this that
a number of elderly living alone have these needs unmet. Since the
chances of living alone greatly increase with age (over 70 percent of
females aged 80 and over are widowed), those elderly most likely to
have health limitations are the ones living alone. We have such common examples as the following:

> Mrs. B. lived in the same house she had lived in for the
> last 40 years. She had five children but they now all had

their own homes, with four living in another state. Mr.
B had died ten years ago. Mrs. B. was now 82. She had
four bedrooms but she only used the one downstairs as
she had trouble climbing stairs. She kept the front par-
lor closed, just using it for the few visitors. Her heating bill was getting too high to heat it. Most of the time
she stayed in the kitchen or the back bedroom. There
was a leak under the kitchen sink but the plumber who
had come last year had not really fixed it. Also the roof
leaked and had stained the walls of one upstairs bedroom,
but she did not use it anyway. The front porch was sagging somewhat and the whole outside needed a coat of
paint, but she hated to go into her small nest egg for the
money; a painter had estimated it would cost $3,000.

Another group of elderly live in boardinghouses and rooming
houses; these 41,000, in many cases, live in transient hotels in inner
city areas or in a private home taking a few elderly boarders, although the definition is such to include supervised boarding arrangements and even some specially designed elderly housing. Some of
these inner city residents are like Mr. K, who lives in a transient
hotel in a skid-row area of San Francisco:

Mr. K. lives in a five-story hotel that was built in 1919.
There are almost 40 rooms; most do not have a separate
bath; the residents are mostly older single men on small
pensions. A few are winos. The floors squeak and the
rooms need painting. On one floor there are still signs
of the fire they had last year when one elderly resident,
smoking in bed, set his mattress on fire. Sometimes
strangers wander into the dingy lobby; one time someone's
check was stolen from his mailbox. The hotel is on a
street with a number of bars and pawnshops. Mr. K.
does not like to walk outside at night. But the room is
cheap, only $70 a month, and his social security check
could not cover a much higher rent.

Housing deprivation is suffered by many inner city elderly, especially the poor elderly. In a 1971 HEW study of elderly on OAA
(now SSI), about 40 percent of the two million OAA elderly surveyed
were living in homes or apartments with substantial physical or structural deficiencies.[16] In a report on Massachusetts housing for the elderly, the authors estimate that most OAA recipients in Boston must
be living in substandard housing; this is based on the fact that the
maximum housing allowance under OAA in 1971 for persons living

alone was $67 a month, and, furthermore, the MIT-Harvard study of
quality of housing done in the same year for the Boston area concluded that, almost without exception, units renting for less than $85
a month in Boston would be considered substandard. The authors add
that "a study of Boston OAA recipients in 1971 by Brandeis University's Gerontological Institute supported this conclusion in general,
though conditions were found to vary with the area of the city."[17]

Of New York City's OAA recipients studied by George Sternlieb,
in his welfare housing study, a large proportion were living in structures built in 1929 or before and a large number were in structures
with a low interior maintenance rating, although on both counts families receiving aid for dependent children were even worse off.[18]

Nationwide, more elderly live in housing without plumbing than
the general population but only 8 percent of the elderly housing lacks
plumbing.[19] Many feel this plumbing criterion does not give a full
picture of the housing condition for the elderly; it ignores such deficiencies as structural condition of the exterior, proper heating and
electrical systems, or fire exits. However, with these limitations,
this gauge does allow us to compare rural and urban, and black and
white, elderly housing status. Almost three times as many rural elderly units as central city elderly units have one or more plumbing
facilities lacking (16 percent for rural units and 5.5 percent for
central city units in standard metropolitan statistical areas). Looking at elderly black households, we find almost one-fourth of them
have inadequate plumbing.[20]

One indication that many elderly are living in deteriorated housing relates to the age of the structure. Well over half, 58 percent,
of elderly owned houses were built before 1939, even though only 36
percent of all owned houses were that old. Elderly renters, usually
living in buildings with fewer than ten units, were even more likely
to live in old structures, even though they moved much more often
than elderly owners. Nearly half of elderly headed owner households
lived in their home for 20 years or more.[21] In this housing overcrowding was not generally a problem, with only 3 percent living in
a unit defined as overcrowded, that is, more than one person to a
room. In fact many elderly overutilize space. In 1962, one study
showed that over half of the elderly surveyed had three or more rooms
per person and another 31 percent had two to three rooms per person.[22]

Housing occupied by elderly suffers from other problems. Due
to size of many units and to their age, heating is a serious problem.
In the study done by HEW of two million OAA recipients, almost half
of them said not every room in their dwelling unit was heated in winter.[23]

In the HAP study many of the allowance recipients said they
did not have adequate heating. Of the recipients who had moved to
standard units, a large group said "inadequate heating" was a problem
before they moved and 23 percent even found it a problem after the
move. For all recipients around a quarter of them found inadequate
heating a problem. In this study elderly satisfaction with their house
seemed related to their satisfaction with the adequacy of their heating.
Half with inadequate heating expressed low satisfaction with the housing.[24]

In the HAP study other problems mentioned by this group of
recipients, who had moved, were connected with rats, leaking roofs,
electrical fuses, and incomplete plumbing. In the Sternlieb study of
welfare recipients, including elderly recipients, almost a third felt
building maintenance and also apartment maintenance was poor, indicating housing deprivation in this area.

Problems of Homeowners

The approximately 70 percent of the elderly living in an owned
unit suffer from several types of housing deprivation. They are living in older structures and, in some cases, substandard structures
lacking adequate plumbing; this is especially true for rural homeowners (and more rural than urban elderly are homeowners), and for
black elderly homeowners (although fewer black than white elderly
are homeowners). A number of the owners (316, 000) own mobile
homes.[25] Many of these units, with age, develop a variety of structural defects.

Maintenance is a major problem for all these elderly. They
live in older structures that are likely to need repairs, whether due
to a leaking roof, a sagging porch, or an unpainted wall. Yet many
of them lack either the funds or the physical strength to make these
repairs. Even routine maintenance such as trimming the shrubs,
mowing the lawn, or repairing a leaking sink, may be too much for
them. This is especially true of older women. In our Canadian study
one of the main reasons for moving to the development was that they
could not maintain their own home anymore; of HAP recipients who
formerly had owned, a reason for selling the house related to inability
to maintain it, and another one was cost of the repairs. While most
of the elderly no longer have mortgages on their homes, their equity
in the house is low, with the 1970 census showing the median equity
for male elderly homeowners at $17, 000.[26] Many banks are reluc-
tant to extend loans to the elderly for house repairs, and a number
of elderly are hesitant to take out a loan on their home both because
they want to pass it on to their children debt free and because they do

not want the loan burden when they are on a fixed income. Some elderly
have received Section 312 grants or loans (see Chapter 4), but this is
a very small proportion of the elderly with maintenance problems.

Elderly homeowners suffer from the problem of increased home
costs, such as in property taxes and insurance, as well as electricity,
heating, and water bill increases. Property taxes have escalated 28
percent between 1963 and 1969; repair costs have gone up a third during this period.[27] Property taxes amounted to 8 percent of income
for all elderly owners in 1970, and were a higher percentage for the
poor elderly.[28] While many states and a number of municipalities
have property tax exemptions for the elderly (see Chapter 4), this by
no means relieves them of the entire tax burden.[29] Even in 1968 it
was concluded in one study that elderly homeowners had an average
housing expenditure of about $600, and those with an income of $5,000
or over had an expenditure of over $900 average.[30] This is likely to
be much higher today, when taxes, insurance, heating, electricity,
water, sewage, and garbage bills are added together; the author's cal-
culations for owner-occupied housing with no mortgage in one rural
area was $150 a month in 1974. Since elderly owners have low incomes,
with 62 percent of all elderly owners in 1970 having family incomes
of less than $5,000,[31] these expenditures for housing, which do not
include repairs and maintenance, represent a considerable financial
burden. On average it is estimated that elderly owners spent at least
one-fifth of their income for essential housing expenditures; for many
it is closer to a fourth, and if they are elderly owners 75 and over it
can be over a fourth, mainly because their income is lower.[32]

The rent burden for elderly renters is considerably higher. Almost half of the elderly renter households in 1970 paid 35 percent or
more of their income for rent. Female elderly renters were in a
worse situation, with almost two-thirds of these women aged 75 and
over, living alone, paying over a third of their income for rent. The
one-person elderly households in general suffered from a high rent-
income burden, with well over half these households paying a third
of their income for rent.[33]

The average 1970 rent for households with an elderly head was
$88; it was higher in suburban areas than in central city, and higher
by far in central city than in rural areas.[34] The amount of rent
paid went up with income. Elderly renters, even more than owners,
are on the losing side of inflation, with no equity in a house and no
chance of selling it at a higher price, but instead the expectation of
higher rents each year. Property tax exemption programs do them
no good. Their only hope may be the expansion of the housing allowance program, or inclusion in the Section 8 program while they stay
in their present residence or move to a qualifying unit.

NOTES

1. James Montgomery, "The Housing Patterns of Older Families," The Family Coordinator 21 (January 1972): 39-41.

2. Ibid.

3. A. S. Cluff and P. J. Cluff, "Design for the Elderly," The Canadian Architect, September 1970, pp. 37-39; M. Powell Lawton, "Planner's Notebook: Planning Environments for Older People," American Institute of Planners Journal, March 1970, pp. 124-29.

4. Research and Development Goals in Social Gerontology; Living Arrangements of Older People: Ecology," The Gerontologist 9 (Winter 1969); 1971 White House Conference on Aging, Housing the Elderly (Washington, D.C.: U.S. Government Printing Office, 1971).

5. National Center for Housing Management, Housing for the Elderly: The On-Site Housing Manager's Resource Book (Washington, D.C.: National Center for Housing Management, 1974), chap. 2, p. 13.

6. Ibid., chap. 8 (devoted to security procedures).

7. Cluff and Cluff, "Design for the Elderly," pp. 36-39.

8. "Research and Development Goals in Social Gerontology; Living Arrangements of Older People: Ecology," p. 41; Lawton, "Planner's Notebook," p. 128, also mentions problems of sharing or roommates.

9. U.S. Department of Housing and Urban Development, Older Americans: Facts about Income and Housing (Washington, D.C.: U.S. Government Printing Office, 1973), p. 48.

10. National Center for Housing Management, Housing for the Elderly, chap. 2, p. 3; from housing production data, U.S. Department of Housing and Urban Development, December 31, 1972; U.S., Congress, Senate, Special Committee on Aging, Adequacy of Federal Response to Housing Needs of Older Americans, Hearings, testimony of Abner Silverman, 94th Cong., 1st sess., October 1975, pt. 14, p. 986.

11. Interview with Anthony Phipps concerning his examination of various directories for housing the elderly, 1975.

12. "Socio-Economic and Housing Characteristics of the Elderly," HUD Challenge 6 (May 1975): 33.

13. U.S. Department of Housing and Urban Development, Older Americans: Facts about Income and Housing.

14. Abraham Monk, "The Emergence of Day Care Centers for the Aged: Trends and Planning Issues" (paper presented at the National Conference on Social Welfare, May 20, 1974).

15. U.S. Department of Commerce, Bureau of the Census, Detailed Characteristics, U.S. Summary: 1970 (Washington, D.C.: U.S. Government Printing Office, 1972), Tables 204, 205.

16. U.S. Congress, Joint Economic Committee, The New Supplementary Security Income Program—Impact on Current Benefits and Unresolved Issues, Joint Committee, Studies in Public Welfare, Paper 10, 93d Cong., 1st sess., 1973; also see U.S. Department of Health, Education and Welfare, Office of Human Development, Administration on Aging, New Facts about Older Americans (Washington, D.C.: U.S. Government Printing Office, June 1973).

17. Barbara Manard, Cary Kart, and Dirk van Gils, Old-Age Institutions (Lexington, Mass.: D. C. Heath, 1974), p. 55.

18. George Sternlieb and Bernard Indik, The Ecology of Welfare: Housing and the Welfare Crisis in New York City (New Brunswick, N.J.: Transaction Books, 1973), pp. 56–58, 75–77.

19. U.S. Department of Housing and Urban Development, Older Americans: Facts about Income and Housing; U.S. Department of Commerce, Bureau of the Census, Housing Characteristics by Household Composition: 1970 (Washington, D.C.: U.S. Government Printing Office, 1973), Tables A–5, B–5, C–5, D–5.

20. Ibid.

21. Ibid., Table A–4.

22. James Morgan, "Measuring the Economic Status of the Aged," cited in 1971 White House Conference on Aging, Housing the Elderly, p. 14.

23. U.S. Department of Health, Education and Welfare, New Facts about Older Americans; also U.S. Congress, Joint Economic Committee, The New Supplemental Security Income Program.

24. Marie McGuire Thompson, Design of Housing for the Elderly (Washington, D.C.: National Association of Housing and Redevelopment Officials, 1972), also stresses the need for heating.

25. U.S. Department of Commerce, Bureau of the Census, Subject Report: Housing of Senior Citizens, 1970 (Washington, D.C.: U.S. Government Printing Office, 1972), HC(7)-2, Tables A–4, A–1.

26. U.S. Department of Commerce, Bureau of the Census, Housing Characteristics by Household Composition: 1970, Tables A–2, B–2, C–2, D–1.

27. 1971 White House Conference on Aging, Housing the Elderly, p. 19.

28. Data from U.S. Department of Commerce, Bureau of the Census, 1970 Residential Finance Survey, and quoted in Financing Schools and Property Tax Relief: A State Responsibility (Washington, D.C.: Advisory Commission on Intergovernmental Relations, December 1972), p. 38.

29. Eady Edsell, "Real Property Tax Relief for the Elderly," Journal of Law Reform, vol. 7 (Winter 1974).

30. Sidney Goldstein, "Home Tenure and Expenditure Patterns of the Aged, 1960–61," The Gerontologist 8 (Spring 1968): 17–24.

31. U.S. Department of Housing and Urban Development, Older Americans: Facts about Income and Housing, p. 30.

32. Goldstein, "Home Tenure and Expenditure Patterns of the Aged," pp. 17–24.

33. U.S. Department of Commerce, Bureau of the Census, Subject Reports: Housing of Senior Citizens, 1970, Table A-4.

34. U.S. Department of Commerce, Bureau of the Census, Housing Characteristics by Household Composition: 1970, Tables A-2, B-2, C-2, D-2.

CHAPTER
4

ASSISTANCE TO THE ELDERLY
IN THEIR OWN HOMES

For the vast majority of the elderly who are still living in their own home, whether an apartment or owner-occupied house, every means should be found to allow them to continue this life style. The elderly cherish this independent living and the privacy it affords them. In their period of life, even more than at earlier periods, the house is their castle, a place of peace and quiet, and a place of happy memories and family photographs and mementos. The home is a focal point—a spatial center for an often more constricted life due to mobility problems.[1] For many of the 70 percent of the elderly who are homeowners, the house is a source of status and of assets.

Of all these features of the home, the fact that it allows independent living is the most important, for it gives a psychological satisfaction. Another type of independence is being able to make the choice between different types of housing arrangements, including one's own home, specially designed apartments, and congregate housing, all readily available. The goal of promoting independence and choice is one that should be incorporated into any housing policy. This is emphasized by Mary Hill, who says there should be

> the provision of as wide a variety and range of choices as possible . . . there should be provisions for a sufficient number of accommodations for those who wish to remain in their own home . . . [there is] need to balance provisions for security with provisions for independence in status for older persons. . . . Another form of balance is to balance between "reaching out" to older people to provide them with a choice of activities and interests on one hand and on the other balancing this with not intruding on their privacy. We know that some elderly lifestyles

require high activity—but we also know that some seniors
show high life satisfaction with a low level of activity.[2]

Different types of assistance are required to improve the quality of
life of these elderly in private housing. It has already been pointed
out that many of these private units the elderly live in are in substandard condition. Some are in transient hotels and housing slated for
demolition. Moreover, many of the units are in deteriorating inner
city neighborhoods and ethnically changing neighborhoods.

The major types of assistance to those in private units are financial assistance to pay their housing bill, rehabilitation expenses in a
few instances, and provision of a variety of supportive services. Financial subsidies differ for renters and owners; they include property
tax exemptions, Section 23 and Section 8 subsidies, SSI overall assistance, and, for a few elderly, the experimental housing allowance.
Supportive services are numerous and include meals on wheels, public health nurse visitations, homemaker services, friendly visiting,
transportation service, and many others.

FINANCIAL ASSISTANCE

For renters, financial assistance can be in terms of some sort
of subsidy for the rent. A very large proportion of the elderly pay
over a third of their income for rent; this can be brought down to 25
percent by government assistance.

At the present time one of the main ways low-income elderly
in private housing can receive financial assistance is through the
leased public housing program, formerly Section 23 and now a new
Section 8. While this usually has required the elderly person to move
to another private unit, a standard one, under contract with the public housing authority, some elderly have received such aid in their
present unit if it is standard and has a rent within specified limits.
Under Section 23 the housing authority usually found the unit, but in
areas where this was difficult due to the low allowable rents limitation
and low vacancy rate, some applicants found their own units.[3] In
some instances the housing authority leased all units in a building,
and those already living there who were eligible came under the program.

This public housing program was a compromise between building
housing for the poor and the other approach, subsidizing the person.
Under the Section 23 leased public housing program, the public housing
authority contracted with a private landlord to lease so many of his
units or his whole building. The housing authority may even have
worked out an arrangement with a developer whereby he built a proj-

ect and then leased units to the housing authority. However, the
project was privately owned and subject to full taxes, unlike conventional public housing. Such a project is the Elms, an elderly project
for 100 households in Secaucus, New Jersey.[4] A leased public housing project, it was designed by architect Arthur Lubetz with the elderly specifically in mind; Marie McGuire Thompson's Design of
Housing for the Elderly was the guide for this building, with its activity areas, court, rooftop garden, reception areas with sun porches
on each floor, and hall railings.[5] Leased public housing can also be
in nonprofit or limited dividend Section 236 housing or Section 202 or
231 housing. For example, the Los Angeles housing authority has
converted a foreclosed Section 231 elderly building, Independent
Square, into leased public housing, taking over management through
a complicated arrangement described in Journal of Housing, July
1975.[6]

Under Section 23 leased public housing, the housing authority
paid the landlord the agreed-upon rent and received from the tenant,
who need not have been elderly, 25 percent of his net income as rent.
While this housing was for low income, with public housing eligibility
levels, some local housing authorities set income limits higher for
Section 23 leased units than for the projects they own.

The program had the characteristics of giving the person assistance in existing units, but they presumably were standard units
found in most cases by the housing authority.

The replacement for Section 23, that is, Section 8, has as an
intent, not an accident, that the applicant search for his own unit. He
or she is given a certificate and then must go out and find housing.
The applicant will negotiate with the landlord, and such matters as
repairs will be a matter between tenant and landlord. The new program prescribes less of a role for the housing authority as adviser
to the tenant and negotiator between tenant and landlord than under
Section 23.[7] Yet in the early stage of this program, it seems authorities are providing information on available units in a number of instances, and some authorities, such as New York City Housing Authority, are finding ingenious ways to locate vacant units; Settlement
Housing Fund, a New York City nonprofit group, has established a
computerized Section 8 housing data bank of potentially suitable and
available apartment units and keeps track of which are becoming vacant.[8]

The housing authority also becomes involved with the applicant,
not only in determining his eligibility and giving him a certificate,
but in explaining to him what constitutes a standard unit, safe, decent, and sanitary, that will be eligible under the program. Since,
for the Section 8 program, HUD has established fair market rents
or maximum rent levels by unit size for each county and metropolitan

area, the local housing authority must also advise the applicant on these levels and possibly work to get HUD's consent to a slightly higher rent (120 percent of established rents).

Since the HUD regional offices have two allocations, one for the Section 8 existing housing program and one for Section 8 new construction/substantial rehabilitation, the housing authority may also be involved in informing applicants about the new units.

The use of new and rehabilitated housing for Section 8 means the regional HUD offices call for bids from developers. In the case of the elderly, 100 percent of the units in the new housing can be rented to low-income elderly. HUD expects that 40 percent of the housing construction under Section 8 will be for the elderly; from present indications it may be much higher. It is assumed that Section 202 housing for the elderly program, and possibly a revived Section 236, will be the programs used by developers to build the units leased under Section 8. The 1974 Housing Act states that housing assistance payments under the new Section 8 program may be used for families in Section 202 projects.

While many housing officials have had trouble making Section 8 work, at the time of this writing (July 1976) over 11,000 units had been processed by one HUD area: 31 northern California housing authorities were participating in the Section 8 existing housing program, and there were 40 northern California projects of new construction/substantial rehabilitation, supplying one-third (almost 3,000) of the 11,000 units.[9] Many of the units in both programs are elderly units. Nationwide, a number of rural and semirural areas are taking part in the Section 8 program. In one area, Dakota County, Minnesota, reports indicate the program is successful with landlords, and local government officials are favorable to it, with the latter happy because it does not concentrate recipients in one area and allows freedom of choice. They feel the program works for all but big families. In some areas of Minnesota the fair rent schedules are too low. Officials say "one of the most difficult parts of the program is educating the applicant during the briefing. The forms and paperwork look overwhelming at first."[10] Another problem they allude to is in the applicant's job of making contact with the landlord. They advise the applicant not to identify the program he is part of over the phone; they urge that contact with the owner be made in person, so that the applicant has "a captive audience" to whom to sell the program; and they teach the applicant how to sell the program. We feel the elderly are less likely to sell the program, and contact by minority elderly may end in subtle rejection by many landlords. Yet these Dakota County housing officials see many good points in the program:

Is Section 8 better? In many respects we found that it is. Not everyone wants to live in a beautiful elderly high rise building. . . . Sometimes the reason is dislocation from familiar neighborhoods; sometimes it is "people-concentration"; sometimes it is fear of heights. Whatever the reason, not all people want to live in the traditional public housing units provided in Dakota County. Section 8 gives people a choice. They do not have to go to a landlord whom we say has agreed to participate in the program. They do not even have to go to someone whom we have on a list. Under Section 8, qualified tenants have freedom of choice, within the limitations of only three requirements: (1) that the building is decent, safe, and sanitary; (2) that it be within the approved rent limits; and (3) that the owner agrees to allow the subsidy to be used. As an LHA [local housing authority], we find these limitations reasonable and comfortable, except in cases of large families. [11]

The leased public housing program has been popular on the West Coast and been used especially for the elderly. This program has been a means to disperse white elderly in existing housing throughout a city. Some elderly who might not want to be placed in a public housing complex can be given housing assistance through this program, without it even being known they are public housing tenants; sometimes they can stay in their present unit. Landlords have been more willing to participate in the program when they are serving elderly who they consider, as tenants, to be better than families. In addition, more small-size private market rent units than large-size units are available in most cities, and thus the available units are the ones best suited to the elderly; in fact residential hotels have in some cases been made available and been converted to efficiency apartments.

San Francisco is one of the cities that has had success with the Section 23 leasing program. In 1969, of San Francisco's 746 leased units, less than 25 percent were located in ghetto areas and over 67 percent were located in lower-income white areas. Over 75 percent of the leased units were occupied by elderly tenants. Norman Peel and Garth Pickett point out that

This may account for the San Francisco Housing Authority's ability to scatter them so widely. Many of the leased units in the more affluent white areas are occupied by the elderly families who occupied them before the units were leased by the housing authority. Such units are often taken over by the housing authority because the elderly tenants can no longer meet the rent; . . . the tenants are normally white

since the area is almost totally white. Fifty-three per
cent of the leased unit tenants are non-white; of these
nearly all are Negro. With most of the units located
in white areas and one-half of the units occupied by Ne-
groes, section 23 housing is the most integrated public
housing program in San Francisco. However, units occupied by elderly tenants make integration easier. [12]

While Section 23 leased public housing has had the advantages
for the elderly of allowing them to live in housing dispersed throughout the city and in anonymous nonstigmatized units, including their
former residence, the program also has had disadvantages. For the
elderly it has meant that in many cases they were not housed in new
units and not in specially designed units that have facilities and design features useful to this particular group, nor are they concentrated in a large complex that can be easily serviced by such community organizations as visiting public health nurses, meal preparation services, or transportation services.

Leased public housing programs are now seriously hampered
by the lack of available units at rents allowed by HUD. At the time
of this writing many housing authorities are trying to substantiate
that they need a higher allowable rent level if they are going to be able
to run a Section 8 program; in some areas they find few units renting
at the HUD listed rents.

A second problem in finding housing at these rents in most cities
is the low vacancy rate at the present time. In the research on elderly
under the housing allowance experimental program, it was found that
in cities where there was a low vacancy rate eligible elderly were
much less likely to use the program.

A third problem single elderly have in utilizing the program relates to HUD's opinion that these elderly should be in efficiency or
studio units, while the elderly themselves want one-bedroom units.
A problem of the housing authority is that of being able to run either
the Section 23 or Section 8 programs under the constraints of the low
administrative operating costs allowed by HUD.

Another program close to a housing allowance and in existence
nationally for both elderly and families has been the rent supplement
program. Unlike a housing allowance, the payments have been limited
to low-income occupants of specially designated, or new or substantially rehabilitated housing—first, under Section 231(d)(3), and then,
236 and 202 nonprofit and limited dividend housing. The supplement
has been paid to the landlord and is tied to the housing unit. The program has subsidized the rent payment of low-income households, with
the government contributing the difference between market rentals
and one-fourth of the household's income after allowable deductions.

Henry Aaron pointed out that the chief innovation of the rent supplement program was that it varied assistance systematically with tenant income in order to focus federal outlays on the poor. As the tenant's income rose, his rent increased until it reached market level; at this point (unlike the situation in public housing) he was not compelled to move but to pay full rent. Aaron pointed out that the program has worked as follows:

> HUD agrees with a contractor to make rent supplement payments at a stipulated maximum per year for forty years. Having secured this commitment, the housing developer then begins construction.
>
> . . . Since some tenants pay more than the basic 30 per cent of market rents, actual payments do not reach the contracted maximum; HUD estimates that over the life of projects authorized from 1967 through 1971, payments were about 83 per cent of the maximum obligation. Rent supplements may be provided for those in housing programs for the elderly and handicapped and for lower income families, in below-market interest rate projects, or in state aided projects.[13]

By the end of 1971, Aaron estimated there were 22,000 rent supplement units completed, many under the Section 236 program, a program whose future ended with the 1973 moratorium. The rent supplement program has not caught on; a very large proportion of the Section 236 projects have had no units under rent supplement. Originally it was decided 20 percent of their units could be under rent supplement; in a few cases a much larger proportion have been under rent supplement.

Tenants in the rent supplement program have been found in general to be very poor. Half the participants were 50 or over in 1969 and almost half were one- or two-person families; the proportion has increased since then.

On top of these, some elderly in their own homes get assistance through the HUD-sponsored experimental housing allowance run in a number of cities, but, before that is detailed, one needs to point out that the largest cash assistance programs to the elderly to assist in their housing expenditures are the SSI payments (formerly OAA) to the poor elderly and the social security (Old-Age Survivors and Disability Insurance) benefits most elderly receive. Over 5 million elderly now receive SSI payments. These recipients, who have overall income maintenance money, have been found in several studies to be unable to use their housing portion of these funds to good advantage. For example, a study by HEW in 1965 of two million elderly then on OAA[14] found 40 percent of these welfare recipients living in housing with substantial physical or structural deficiencies, with the percentage of poor elderly running as high as 70 percent in bad housing in rural and southern areas. In a New York City study done by Sternlieb, many SSI recipients were found to be living in older buildings with low maintenance ratings.

These SSI and social security checks are of course assistance to the person. Another one, specially for housing and called a housing allowance, is being experimented with in eight medium-size cities in the United States under HUD funding. Over 2000 poor elderly are taking part in this experiment; they receive assistance to fill the gap between the rent they must pay and 25 percent of their income. Many of these elderly recipients have been able to stay in their own units, according to the HUD-sponsored study (noted previously) that the author took part in; others have had to move to meet the criterion of living in a standard unit.

The program is nearer a true housing allowance approach, as found in Europe,[15] than the case of the Section 8 program but is similar to Section 8. After applying to the administrative agency and being qualified according to income eligibility regulations, the person gets a certificate saying he is eligible, and then he searches for housing. He does the hunting and negotiating with the landlord himself, although the different agencies participating in this experiment give different degrees and different variations of counseling to the applicant. The information, of course, includes explanation of the program and the applicant's role but it may also include guidelines on how to hunt for a unit, sometimes information on apartment availability or likely areas of available apartments, guidelines on how to determine whether the apartment is standard and what the criteria for standardness are, as well as information on lease negotiation techniques and occasionally on affirmative action and eviction regulations.

The reimbursement to the recipient is determined by a payment formula based on a support level approximating a reasonable housing cost for a given household size for that area (contract rent level set for each area), minus 25 percent of the net household income.[16] Formulas differed somewhat with different experiment locales.

The first of these experiments, prior to the HUD-sponsored ones, was the small OEO Kansas City, Missouri, experiment, which Arthur Solomon's MIT group has studied. The HUD-sponsored larger experiments have been the demand-side experiments run in Pittsburgh and Phoenix, and the administrative agency experiments run in eight medium-size cities or areas, including Springfield, Massachusetts; Tulsa, Oklahoma; Durham, North Carolina; Peoria, Illinois; Salem, Oregon; San Bernardino County, California; Bismarck, North

Dakota; and Jacksonville, Florida. Abt Associates has been conducting both these sets of experiments and did a special survey of elderly applicants and recipients in the eight cities and areas under the administrative agency experiment. Rand Corporation is running the supply experiment in two Midwest cities.

Evidence from research on these experimental housing allowance programs shows this type of financial assistance can be helpful to the elderly;[17] the programs reach people who need monetary assistance with their housing bill, but might not want to apply for welfare (SSI). The majority of elderly surveyed in the administrative agency experiment were not on SSI. In some cases, these elderly also benefit from counseling on available units and from encouragement on various aspects of the moving process. Through the programs, a number of them had their housing quality and neighborhood quality improved because they had to move to standard housing.

For example, Solomon[18] reports that in the Kansas City OEO housing allowance experiment the recipients, all living in a very deteriorated slum area, moved to new neighborhoods of higher socioeconomic status in terms of median family income, educational level, and occupation of head of household; 58 percent of the families moved completely out of the 1970 census-defined poverty areas. They moved to areas with a higher proportion of owner-occupied units, higher rents, lower density, and lower crime rates. They moved to fringe city areas but not suburbs.

Of the surveyed elderly in the administrative agency housing allowance experiment, many did not move as they were usually already in a standard unit, but of those who did move to standard housing to take part in the experiment, a majority changed neighborhoods. Many movers were more satisfied with their neighborhood, in terms of transportation availability and safeness from crime, than other groups in the sample, especially those who tried to move and failed to find a unit.

Those who did move after enrolling in the housing allowance program in most cases showed an improved situation over their former housing, with the great majority of those lacking one of the three basic facilities (adequate heat, complete kitchen, and piped water) before they moved now being in housing that had all three facilities. Before they moved almost a third had been in housing lacking complete plumbing; almost half had had poor heating; almost a third had had mice or rats; over a third had had a leaking roof or ceiling; a fifth had not had hot water. After the move most of these recipients were now living in standard units, often single-family dwellings; very few said there were problems with hot water, with plumbing, and with incomplete kitchen, though some still said they had problems of inadequate heating in their new unit, leaking roof, and problems with rats. These movers were far more satisfied with their housing unit than those that had tried to move, usually to qualify for the program, but been unsuccessful in moving.[19]

The elderly applicants who wanted to move to take part in the program but did not, seemed most worried about having money for a security deposit and moving expenses; some were concerned about negotiating a lease, which many had never done before, and about inspecting the unit for standardness as well as obtaining transportation to do this inspecting. For such a program to succeed, many will need help in a number of areas, such as information on available units and where they are located, including how close they are to public transportation and shopping. These elderly applicants will need help on judging whether a unit is standard and whether it has the physical design features important to them, such as adequate heating, and an elevator and lack of stairs. They will need help on security deposits and moving expenses. They need to know about applicable affirmative action regulations, lease negotiations, and eviction procedure.

These surveyed elderly interested in the housing allowance program have all said that, to participate, there must be a unit they can afford in a neighborhood they desire. This is a wish also held, one feels, by Section 8 applicants. This is a problem when it is a low-vacancy-rate and high-rent area, because these types of financial assistance programs place limits on the rents that can be paid, even though the maximum rents are determined by area. These programs, according to early indications, work best in cities where there is a high vacancy rate and a high degree of standard housing available at moderate rents. Reports indicate in cities where there is a low vacancy rate and low quality of housing stock, many applicants who want to participate in the program may have trouble doing so, whether it is an experimental housing allowance program or the Section 8 program. In one medium-size city where the housing allowance program worked well, with many elderly moving to standard units, and a lower enrollee dropout and lower termination rate, there was a fairly high vacancy rate for applicable apartments, a very low substandard rate, low rents, few lease requirements, and no major housing discrimination problem because the population was mainly white. But there are many areas where the opposite situation exists, with few standard units available at low rents. In this survey of elderly housing allowance participants, many of those who wanted to move and failed did extensive hunting, with a number looking at five or more places. Their main problem was they could not find a place they could afford. And, of course, if many low-income elderly should try to use these programs, the competition for standard units at moderate rents will make it harder to find such and possibly push up the price of these units, defeating the purpose of this financial assistance.

From the supply experiment in two cities, HUD hopes to be able to predict how serious this problem will be. It is already the problem existing for elderly getting SSI, the biggest financial assistance program of all for helping the elderly with their housing bill. Under that grant, one is not limited to living in a standard unit and thus has a wider market, although in some cities recipients mainly have substandard units to choose from.

FINANCIAL ASSISTANCE TO ELDERLY OWNERS

Two types of assistance to homeowners (70 percent of all elderly households) are property tax relief programs and rehabilitation grants and loans. Since many elderly own homes in deteriorating inner city areas that have been designated as conservation areas or, in former days, as code enforcement (FACE) areas, some have benefited from rehabilitation loans at below market interest rates or, if they have low income, from grants, under the Section 312 or other rehabilitation programs.[20]

Rehabilitation programs now are also funded by HUD community development block-grants[21] or local bond issue funding such as in San Francisco, as well as Section 312.

Elderly owners, finding themselves in code enforcement or conservation areas, sometimes have had mixed interest in taking part in the program even though their homes may be in major need of repairs. Many elderly owners do not feel they want to take out loans, even at below market interest rates, at their advanced age; they may not be able to meet even these low loan payments. Some, of course, have income low enough to have qualified for grants under the federal programs, but many others have incomes slightly above the allowable maximum.

Property tax relief programs are another means by which the many elderly owners can get financial assistance toward their housing costs. At the close of 1974, 48 states and the District of Columbia had authorized 83 different programs; the elderly received preferential treatment in all but three of the programs, according to Abt Associates, which did a study of these programs. In many states the programs are basically aimed at the elderly. The circuit breaker program type in 1974 disbursed nearly $500 million in beneifts to 3.2 million claimants, many of them elderly, with an average relief payment of $143, according to the Abt report. They also state that homestead exemptions, the other major program type, distributed in 1973 more than $1 billion in benefits to at least 6.3 million claimants, again many being elderly, with the average benefit standing at $173. These average payments are quite modest, but some state programs make considerably higher payments.[22]

The existing property tax relief programs have as one objective that of enabling the elderly to retain their homes. The other objectives include, according to the Abt report, reducing the regressivity of the property tax, shielding low-income households from large tax liabilities, and slowing neighborhood deterioration. Since property taxes are increasing at fast rates in some areas, any help in paying this bill is appreciated. Most elderly have paid their mortgage off but in 1976 find themselves paying as much as $1,500 to $2,000 a year in property taxes in urban areas. The relief programs are needed, but the question is whether the amount of payment is high enough to be of real use, and whether, in states using a maximum income for cutoff of exemptions, the amount is high enough. In California the income the elderly person can receive and still qualify for senior citizen property tax relief was $4,000 in 1976 but was being raised to $5,000. This California property exemption for qualified persons 62 years or older was also being increased in 1976, to a maximum 96 percent of the first $8,500 of assessed valuation instead of the current $7,500.[23] The anticipated changes included an elderly renter credit as large as $220 in addition to the current $37 credit now in effect.

SUPPORTIVE SERVICES TO HELP THE ELDERLY
STAY IN THEIR OWN HOMES

Decent shelter for reasonable financial outlay is not the only thing the elderly need, as we pointed out in Chapter 2. The elderly often must have assistance with housework and maintenance, with cooking, with transportation problems, and above all with medical problems. They also need social work counseling, recreational opportunities, and social contact services. And, of course, they need information and referral assistance to help them locate all the above aids as well as sources of financial assistance.

A brief description of these services may be useful. Several services may be supplied by one agency and, of course, the same service may be provided by several agencies. The service may be available to only a certain category of elderly, whether those of particular health status, socioeconomic level, or religious or social club affiliation. In some cases the service is a means-tested one available only to low-income elderly, and in others a universal service available to all. Local committees or councils on aging, under Title III of the Older Americans Act, are now trying to coordinate these services, cut down on duplication, and act as the major information and referral source for elderly in the area; these councils also supplement the present programs with needed services and often

have under their domain the coordination and administration of the
Title VII meals-nutrition program. In many areas senior citizen
clubs or centers also take on this role of information and referral
and of instigating new programs.

Because elderly need continued social interaction with others
and cultural and mental stimulation, senior citizen centers can play
an important role. Many centers, besides running the normal recreational program, having tours and special events, now run special
programs for the more passive and the frail elderly. Some centers,
such as in San Francisco,[24] have outreach programs to make contact with the more isolated elderly. Bellevue Hospital in New York
City has had a storefront program for frail elderly in one neighborhood of the city where there is a heavy concentration of elderly.[25]

Many other groups of course run recreational programs for the
elderly, including many city parks and recreation departments,
church groups, and neigborhood groups.

Other social contact services found in many cities are the
friendly visitor program, whereby volunteers call weekly, or on some
regular basis visit elderly who are identified as isolated or somewhat
nonambulatory and in need of contact; in some areas the Red Cross
runs these. This friendly visitor provides not only a social contact
but an aid who acts as a driver who can pick up drug prescriptions
or groceries and, above all, be alerted to any medical problems or
emergency. In fact this volunteer, through weekly contact with the
person, can watch for medical problems and alert the necessary resources or get the person to a health clinic or similar facility. The
telephone contact service is a similar volunteer program, possibly
on a daily basis, where again there is a chance to check up on the
elderly person's health condition. One in the Bay Area, run by a
hospital, is called Tele-Care and is a daily checkup.

A professional visitor is the public health nurse, or a nurse
supplied by some other agency, who may temporarily or on a permanent basis visit elderly who have some health problem, but, with
this care, have the ability to stay in their own home. This nurse
can give medications and shots, take blood pressure, give the person
a bath, take care of podiatry needs, or perform other needed services.

A homemaker service is another type of assistance that can be
offered to a person who has just returned from the hospital, or per-
manently has trouble doing housework, making beds, cooking; the
help may be daily or weekly. The charges may be a sliding scale.
Like all these services, the number of available homemakers is small
compared to the degree of need (see Table 4.1).

The elderly person having trouble with food preparation, including widowers, can also turn to a meals-on-wheels service, whereby
volunteers deliver a noon meal available through an agency, service

TABLE 4.1

Difficulty with Housework, Cooking, and Shopping

Area of Difficulty	Yes, Has Difficulty	No Difficulty	No Answer	Total
Housework				
Number	91	199	13	303
Percent	30.0	65.7	4.3	100
Cooking				
Number	67	192	44	303
Percent	22.2	63.4	14.5	100
Shopping in winter				
Number	107	179	17	303
Percent	35.3	59.0	5.6	100

Source: Canadian user survey.

club, or church group program. The volunteer also fills the same role as the friendly visitor but on a more frequent basis. Some elderly do not care for the program, either because the food is not to their liking or arrives cold. An alternative is for the elderly person to go to a neighborhood senior meals program, which is now found in many areas under Title VII assistance (see Chapter 6 for details). This is better for ambulatory elderly as it gets them out of the house once a day and gives them a chance to socialize with other elderly and take advantage of other programs run in the same center.

In a few cities, in areas where there is a concentration of elderly, medical clinics especially catering to elderly needs have been established. Elderly in the area of a hospital might get preferential treatment there.

Special transportation services are often available from the city or some agency to take the elderly to community services, to shopping facilities, and to church. In some cases these are minibuses run on a regular basis or on a phone-in basis. In some places, taxi costs for such trips by the elderly are covered by the agency. For example, the Alameda County, California, Office on Aging has made this one of their special projects and, in cooperation with some cities of the county, gives special transportation assistance, using the different methods described above.

There are a variety of other services run in different cities. For example in several areas, the city or an agency provides minor maintenance assistance to elderly homeowners. All these supportive services can be useful in providing the minor assistance needed for many elderly to stay in their own homes and live an independent life.

A last service to mention are the day care programs now being started in many cities. These programs are of a different nature than the above in that they are directed at impaired elderly who have only a marginal degree of competence, while the above programs are directed at ambulatory, or in a few cases, semiambulatory, elderly who are still quite competent. The day care program in a number of cases serves elderly persons that live in their adult children's home, although some do live in their own home, possibly with a spouse, sibling, or adult child present to care for their needs. This program is a substitute for the nursing home. The clientele, researchers report, are "those individuals whose mental and/or physical health no longer allows them to remain in the community unless they have the support of a family (or surrogate family) and the structure of a day care setting. Without these support factors they would be at the risk of institutionalization."[26] A day care program takes the burden of caring for the elderly person off the hands of relatives for a good part of the day. At the same time it allows the elderly person to get the enjoyment of being with his or her family in the evenings and on weekends instead of being relegated to the institutional setting of the nursing home. Day care programs are, of course, also much less costly than nursing homes.[27]

The types of needs these day care programs serve, and the type of elderly utilizing them, may differ from program to program. Some are run by hospitals or nursing homes such as the Levindale Hebrew Geriatric Center and Hospital in Baltimore.[28] Abraham Monk[29] reports they are also housed in multiservice senior centers, rehabilitation centers, homes for the aged, and even social service departments. He adds that most centers serve at the most 15 to 20 elderly and he gives, as the main sources of financing in 1974, Medicaid and Title III of the Older Americans Act.

Eloise Rathbone-McCuan and Julia Levenson, reporting on these day care programs, say, "participation in an institutionally based day care center can be defined as a 'marginal' form of institutionalization. It can be conceived of as a setting in which aged people spend a portion of their time and receive an array of services without forfeiting the option of living in the community."[30] They add that day care participants have some home setting where they spend the greatest part of their time, even though they may be in the center eight hours a day, five days a week.

E. Robins has defined these day care programs in detail:

Day care is a program of services provided under health leadership in an ambulatory care setting for adults who do not require 24-hour institutional care and yet, due to physical and/or mental impairment, are not capable of full-time independent living. Participants are referred to the program by their attending physician or by some other appropriate sources such as an institutional discharge planning program, a social service agency, etc. The essential elements of a day care program are directed toward meeting the health maintenance and restoration needs of participants. However, there are socialization elements in the program.[31]

At the Levindale day care center,[32] serving 30 elderly, their staff includes a nurse, a social worker, an aide, an orderly, an occupational therapist, a physical therapist, a recreation therapist, and transportation drivers. Health-related services include medication, modified exercise, and dressings and treatments, all taken care of directly by the staff, and then, available through inpatient resources of the hospital, chiropody, and occupational and physical and speech therapy. Bathing and dietary services are also provided, plus an extensive range of recreational programs.

This center has more services staff than many of the 18 nationwide centers Monk surveyed.[33] He found recreation was a common denominator in all centers, but almost all provided counseling, social services, and meals, though less than a third included physical, occupational, and remotivational therapy. Another third—five—did not offer any of these and just four included medical service for ambulatory patients who are chronically ill. As the number of these centers increases and their potential as alternatives to the nursing home is recognized, the number of services offered may grow.

The usual routine for these centers is for a driver to pick up the elderly person at the person's home or the person's family's home. This may include helping the person to complete dressing, to lead him or wheel his wheelchair to a van, and get him in. The provision of this transportation service is essential to the program and a time-consuming process. Often a number of trips to different areas of the city need to be made. The program, Monk reports,[34] usually runs from 9 a.m. or 10 a.m. to 2:30 or 4 p.m. After arrival, there is a coffee and socialization time; organized activity such as arts and crafts, lectures, discussion groups, games, films, music; individualized rehabilitation such as exercise, physical therapy, and counseling; a hot meal at noon followed by a rest period, then recreational and rehabilitative programs. Monk found most centers operated five days a week; only two of his 18, seven days; and three had vacation care.

The next chapter shows another type of solution in meeting these needs, that is, specially designed apartments and congregate housing for the elderly.

NOTES

1. Elizabeth D. Huttman, "Public Housing: Negative Psychological Effects on Family Living," Journal of American Orthopsychiatric Association 42, no. 2 (March 1971): 165.

2. Mary Hill, "The Quality of Living in Housing for the Elderly," in Proceedings, SPARC conference (Vancouver: SPARC, 1974), pp. 3-4.

3. There has been very little research on Section 23. Most of the data presented here are from oral presentations at meetings of the National Association of Housing and Redevelopment Officials (NAHRO), and talks with local housing authority officials. Also Robert Taggart, Low Income Housing: A Critique of Federal Aid (Baltimore: Johns Hopkins University Press, 1970), covers many of these programs.

4. "Elderly-Oriented Design Creates Cheerful, Bustling Community for Tenants of Secaucus Section 23 Project," Journal of Housing 32 (October 1975): 448-49.

5. Ibid; Marie McGuire Thompson, Design of Housing for the Elderly (Washington, D.C.: National Association of Housing and Urban Redevelopment Officials, 1972).

6. Michael H. Salzman, "Foreclosed Building Redeemed Converted to Leased Housing for Elderly by Efforts, Ingenuity of Los Angeles Housing Authority, Journal of Housing 32 (July 1975): 327-29.

7. "A New HAP Program—A Housing Assistance Payments Program for Lower Income Families," Journal of Housing 31 (August 1974): 354-55.

8. "New York Uses Computers to Locate Section 8 Units," Journal of Housing 33 (May 1976): 235.

9. "Section 8 Update," Pacific Southwest NAHRO News 14 (July 1976): 2.

10. Nan McKay, "Section 8 Is Working Well in Dakota County, Minnesota," Journal of Housing (June 1976): 272-73.

11. Ibid.

12. Norman Peel, Garth Pickett, and Stephen Buehl, "Racial Discrimination in Public Housing Site Selection," Stanford Law Review 23 (November 1970): 66-147.

13. Henry Aaron, Shelter and Subsidies: Who Benefits from Federal Housing Policies? (Washington, D.C.: Brookings Instituttion, 1972), pp. 133-35.

14. U.S. Congress, Joint Economic Committee, The New Supplemental Security Income Program—Impact on Current Benefits and Unresolved Issues, Joint Committee, Studies in Public Welfare, Paper 10, 93d Cong., 1st sess., 1973.

15. Interviews with national and local housing officials administering housing allowance programs in the Netherlands and Sweden, 1968, 1970, 1971.

16. U.S. Department of Housing and Urban Development, Office of Policy Evaluation and Research, First Annual Report of the Experimental Housing Allowance (Washington, D.C.: U.S. Government Printing Office, May 1973).

17. These comments are impressions gained by the author in talking to both HUD officials and administrating personnel, and analysis of survey data on participating elderly. Comments are not given as conclusions of any Abt personnel.

18. Arthur Solomon, Evaluation of the OEO Kansas City Housing Experience (Cambridge: Massachusetts Institute of Technology Press, 1974).

19. Interviews with HUD officials and administrating personnel, and analysis of survey data on participating elderly.

20. Taggart, Low Income Housing, p. 151; George Sternlieb, "Abandonment and Rehabilitation: What Is to Be Done?" in Housing: 1970-1971, ed. George Sternlieb (New York: AMS Press, 1972), pp. 64, 68-72. Sternlieb says the elderly are the weakest of the core housing owners. Their capacity and interest in reinvestment is minimal. They have a horror of assuming a mortgage for rehabilitation.

21. Pat W. Collins, "Community Development Funds Used to Set up Local Rehabilitation Loan Program," Journal of Housing (June 1976): 266-68.

22. Abt Associates, Property Tax Relief Programs for the Elderly, Final report (Washington, D.C.: U.S. Government Printing Office, 1976), p. 3.

23. "Tax Aid Bill for Elderly Gets an OK," San Francisco Chronicle, August 17, 1976, p. 10.

24. Interview with William Pothier, director, San Francisco senior citizen centers, October 1975.

25. Janet Sillen et al., "A Multi-Disciplinary Geriatric Unit for the Psychiatrically Impaired in Bellevue Hospital Center" (paper presented at the American Orthopsychiatric Association meetings, San Francisco, 1975).

26. Eloise Rathbone-McCuan and Julia Levenson, "Impact of Socialization Therapy in a Geriatric Day Care Setting" (paper presented at Gerontological Society meeting, Portland, Oregon, October 1974), p. 3.

27. Abraham Monk, "The Emergence of Day Care Centers for the Aged: Trends and Planning Issues" (paper presented at National Conference on Social Welfare, Cincinnati, May 1975), p. 5.

28. Rathbone-McCuan and Levenson, "Impact of Socialization Therapy."

29. Monk, "The Emergence of Day Care Centers for the Aged," p. 4.

30. Rathbone-McCuan and Levenson, "Impact of Socialization on Therapy," p. 5.

31. E. Robins, "Therapeutic Day Care: Progress Report on Experiments to Test the Feasibility for Third Party Payment" (paper presented at Gerontological Society meeting, Portland, Oregon, October 1974).

32. Rathbone-McCuan and Levenson, "Impact of Socialization on Therapy," p. 3.

33. Monk, "The Emergence of Day Care Centers for the Aged," p. 5.

34. Ibid., pp. 5-6.

5

SPECIALLY DESIGNED APARTMENTS
AND CONGREGATE HOUSING
FOR THE ELDERLY

Elderly, especially those in their mid-seventies, may find living in their own home no longer meets their needs, and their housing requirements would better be filled in specially designed apartments or congregate housing. These elderly want to live as independent a life as possible but they would like relief from some of the burdens they must cope with in their present housing; then, some need a cheaper unit. Their house may be too big to maintain, both in exterior and interior work, and too costly to keep up. It is likely too large and possibly rather old and deteriorated. These elderly would like a small modern unit that would be easy to clean. They would like a unit where exterior maintenance is in the hands of management.

Many older elderly want a complex that has design features that mean less exertion in their old age. They or their family may desire housing with special facilities that cater to their social and physical needs, such as a recreation room and even an infirmary. They may want the companionship of other elderly and the social activities often afforded in such a setting. They want the presence of a cooperative staff they can turn to if there are emergency health needs, and they want another type of security: well-lighted, protected building safe from intruders.

In our Canadian survey the elderly gave all these reasons for coming to specially designed elderly housing developments, as shown in Table 3.1.

A majority coming to specially designed complexes want an apartment where they can still cook and live a fully independent life. However, for some impaired but not ill elderly, a more supportive or sheltered environment, with dining room meals, possibly housekeep-

ing assistance, and even some nursing staff, may be needed. Such
a supportive environment will allow these elderly to get about on their
own; at the same time it provides backup services to cover their deficiencies. These elderly, even more than those moving into apartments, are at the point in their physical and possibly mental deterioration where staying in their own home is not an asset but a case
of serious lack of needed help, a case where a person is not getting
adequate meals or keeping a house clean and possibly not receiving
needed medical-nursing care.

Speaking in 1975 before the Senate Special Committee on Aging,
of the need for an alternative to the elderly person's own home, Wilma
Donahue said: "It has been amply demonstrated that there is need for
specially designed housing with a variety of associated services for
scores, if not hundreds of thousands of older people who must now
live under growing apprehension of having too soon to seek refuge in
long-term medical care facilities as they progress through the later
years of their lives. These are the impaired but not ill, non-insti-
tutionalized, often low-income older people who must struggle against
rising odds to maintain themselves in the community." Donahue
pointed out that "assisted residential living, especially congregate
housing, would extend significantly the period of time impaired though
not ill older people are able to remain in the community enjoying the
independence, autonomy, privacy, and social relationships that constitute the very essence of meaningful life." She added that "family
members, vitally concerned with the well-being of older relatives,
would be relieved of most of the sometimes overwhelming burden of
trying to provide continuing assistance to them and of the extreme
sense of guilt usually associated with consigning aged parents to a
nursing home from which few return."[1]

In this chapter we discuss both types of specially designed
housing, apartments and congregate arrangements, even though we
realize the congregate complexes, because they serve elderly with
more health problems and less ability to live independently, have
more supportive services and facilities than apartments. However,
because there is such an overlap in services and in design features
for the two and because many developments have both apartments and
congregate wings, with dining facilities, we feel it is better, after an
introduction making distinctions between the two, to discuss them
jointly in the rest of the chapter.

SPECIALLY DESIGNED APARTMENTS AND
RETIREMENT COMMUNITIES

Specially designed apartments and retirement communities can
take a number of forms. Many are public housing complexes; there

were 273,270 such specially designed elderly public housing units as
of 1975 (there were a half million units occupied by elderly in January
1975 but the rest were in mixed projects).[2] Specially designed developments can also be the somewhat more expensive nonprofit or limited
dividend projects under Section 202/236; there were around 100,000
of these as of 1975.[3] However, over 60 percent of the Section 202
projects in 1972 had dining rooms; there were also some luxurious
Section 231 apartment units, although most of these also have dining
facilities and thus are congregate housing. One should also mention
the retirement communities, especially in California, Florida, and
the Southwest. These often have small single-family units in cluster-
type arrangement, with a variety of recreational facilities such as
golf courses and community centers; Leisure World is a good example. The units are often owned and there is a monthly maintenance-
service charge; they are mainly financially obtainable to the upper
middle class.

These specially designed elderly apartments or cluster housing
complexes all have in common that they house mainly elderly, though
age limitations may vary, and that their units are designed to meet
the physical needs of this group. The development units have complete kitchens, and the developments usually have special facilities
such as a communal room, reception area-lounge, laundromat, and
possibly one or two offices for visiting or development personnel.
Luxury apartments may, in individual cases, have other types of facilities mentioned below. The range of facilities is usually smaller
than that found in congregate developments. For example, in the
Canadian nonprofit and public housing developments for the elderly,
the typical apartment complex had only a central recreational room
(72 percent had this) and a laundry room (91 percent had this). About
a fifth had a card and game room and 17 percent had a library; 14
percent had a coffee room.

In the United States many elderly public housing complexes now
have a communal room and possibly an office; some have a dining
area where outside groups serve a noon meal. Most have a laundromat. The Los Angeles Housing Authority has one leased housing complex with a library, music room, dining room, meditation room, fun
room, so furnished because it is a former luxury Section 231 development converted to leased housing after financial failure.[4] Many Section 236 developments have a wide array of facilities. Western Park,
a Satellite Homes apartment complex in San Francisco, has lounges,
hobby rooms, and a laundry room. It has a noon hot meals service
for those who want it.[5]

The specially designed apartment complex has, to varying degrees, services of use to ambulatory elderly; however, many are
provided by the community and not the development. Exceptions will

be mentioned in the discussion on services. Many public housing authorities in the United States have a community services division that works with all the elderly public housing developments in its jurisdiction and tries to get activities going, as well as contract with community agencies for services. The most common management-initiated services are in the realm of encouraging or sponsoring tenant recreational activities, organizing tenant clubs or associations, or, as found in our Canadian study, encouraging friendly visiting, telephone contact service, and voluntary transportation assistance. In many authorities the vigor of the effort is erratic and services may exist more on paper than in reality.

Lawton found in 1971 that only a quarter of the public housing developments he surveyed had any on-site medical services; they rarely had a dispensary and dependable on-call emergency service. As for meal service, he found less than a fifth had any meal service. [6] In a later report a HUD official says 700 sites in 400 authorities are using the meal service of the Administration on Aging (AOA) nutrition program. [7] Some Section 202/236 apartment housing also is the site for this one-meal-a-day service, such as Satellite Central in Oakland.

The specially designed apartment complexes usually have less staff than the congregate developments. In some, staff is limited to maintenance personnel with only an area manager. Others, especially nonprofit housing, have managerial staff that, among its many jobs, can meet social needs. Additional staff can include live-in paraprofessionals or students. For example, the public housing authority in San Francisco had live-in couples. Such staff can take care of medical emergencies.

The residents of the apartment developments, when compared with those in congregate developments, differ on several characteristics. They are usually younger than the congregate housing population. For example, in our Canada survey of users, only 10 percent of the apartment residents were 80 or over while almost half of the congregate housing residents were 80 or over. In the United States the median age in public housing apartments especially for the elderly is 72 for females and 69 for males. Just because they are an older group, congregate housing residents are more likely to be widows and to be female, while apartment dwellers include more couples and more men. Yet many apartment dwellers are also widows, for many come to this elderly housing after their spouse has died or when they have developed physical limitations, meaning most are over 70 rather than in the 65-70 group. Only a fifth of our Canadian surveyed users were under 70; over half of the apartment dwellers were living alone.

In retirement cluster housing complexes, such as Leisure World, the age of entry seems to be younger. Hamovitch found in the

southern California retirement community he studied that the mean
age was 66 and that 8 percent were below age 65. The emphasis on
recreational activities, such as golf, in these retirement communities would indicate they attract a younger elderly group.

The socioeconomic level of residents is of course determined
by the type of specially designed housing, with retirement communities of course attracting middle income.* Section 231 housing, mainl
congregate complexes, has also been for the upper middle class.
While Section 236 and Section 202 nonprofit and limited dividend
housing has been considered subsidized housing for the moderate-
income elderly, this housing has in reality served mainly the elderly
near the top allowable income limits; Robert Taggart in 1970 reported
that only 30 percent of the Section 202 housing residents had incomes
below the poverty level, and Irving Welfeld reports that, in general,
Section 236 residents have incomes near the maximum allowable income. [8] It is true that some elderly in Section 236 housing benefited
from the rent supplement program, which reduced their rent payment
to 25 percent of their income, but not many received this supplement;
only 5 percent of all tenants in 1969 were on rent supplement. [9] In the
future, Section 202 should also serve low income.

Public housing of course does serve the low-income elderly;
these elderly households in 1974 had an annual income of $2,624. [10]
In the Canadian study almost half the surveyed public housing elderly
tenants had only their government pension and supplementary benefit;
half felt they had a financial strain on their limited monetary resources.

An interesting irony is that these specially designed apartment
complexes are more available to the low-income elderly than to any
other group, with the upper-middle-income group second most likely
to have such complexes available to them. As already mentioned,
there are almost 300,000 specially designed public housing elderly
units. With well over half of the new Section 8 developments at this
time being developments planned for the elderly, we can assume this
number will increase. Less than 100,000 Section 202/236 units have
been built; many are congregate housing, as is Section 231 housing.
We have no accurate count of the private specially designed elderly
apartment or retirement community complexes for mainly upper-
middle-class elderly but we believe it is far below the third-of-a-
million specially designed public housing units for the elderly.

Healthwise, elderly in these specially designed apartments are
slightly more likely to have physical problems than the elderly popu-

---

*Hamovitch found in his southern California retirement commu-
nity that about one-third were in social classes (SES) 2, 3, and 4,
and almost none in social classes 5 or 1.

lation in general, though our information is mainly on public housing residents. In our Canadian study, apartment dwellers in public housing and nonprofit housing themselves said they had "slightly limited ability." Only a tenth had "moderately" or "seriously" limited ability. Interviewers' assessments were that 31 percent were somewhat infirm and 3 percent obviously ill or infirm. In the separate survey of managers, nine out of every ten of these apartment development managers said the average degree of incapacity of their residents was "no incapacity." Almost two-thirds said they had no residents with "moderate" or with "seriously" limited ability. In contrast to this situation, many residents of congregate housing did have fairly serious health problems, as detailed below.

In U.S. public housing, many elderly have been found to have some health limitations even if only minor ones. Lawton reports that in his 1971 research on 2,000 public housing tenants, two-thirds of these interviewed tenants expressed the need for some security-giving on-site medical service; he adds that there was a very high level of support for the availability of assistance with housekeeping and personal care. [11] Donahue reports from studying public housing tenants that many said they had limited mobility and others mentioned frailty, chronic disease, crippling arthritis, visual impairment, and mental confusion, in that order. Donahue also reports that the survey indicates that 12.3 percent of elderly persons in public housing need more assistance than is currently available to them. [12]

In fact, there is presently a crisis in public housing for the elderly because many residents have a degree of physical disability that means they need supportive services. Marie McGuire Thompson reports:

> Many tenants now in public housing have "aged" in their present quarters as have those in private housing in the community. As could be anticipated, an increasing number of public housing agencies are faced with the fact that either they must evict the more frail or impaired who cannot sustain the shopping, cooking, or heavy housekeeping chores designed for the hale and hearty, or they must develop on a crash, and, perhaps, ill-founded basis—some semblance of the services these aging occupants need to maintain at least semi-independence in a residential setting. [13]

Donahue reports that in her survey of public housing authorities she found that many directors, when asked, felt they had a need for a congregate housing wing or project. One director said: "Every year, a large number of our tenants must leave our elderly housing

projects and go into nursing homes. I am convinced that if we had
a congregate housing project under management, that we could extend the number of years of independent living for our elderly tenants."[1]

Another housing official told Donahue: "There seems to be no
program available to our authority . . . but there is certainly need
for a congregate facility. One of our biggest problems is how to make
arrangements for those needing services we cannot provide."

CONGREGATE HOUSING

Congregate housing is considered to meet these needs. Congregate housing usually includes a dining room where three meals a day
are served and various supportive services offered. In many there
is a hotel-type bedroom rather than a fully equipped apartment.
There are usually numerous facilities. It is considered housing for
ambulatory elderly who can walk to their meals and do not need major
nursing care.

The International Center for Social Gerontology has defined
congregate housing as "a residential environment which includes services, such as meals, housekeeping, health, personal hygiene, and
transportation, which are required to assist impaired, but not ill,
elderly tenants to maintain or return to a semiindependent life style
and avoid institutionalization as they grow older."[15]

The HUD official definition of congregate housing used in the
1970 Housing and Urban Development Act and in the 1974 Housing and
Community Development Act is, low-cost housing in which some or all
dwelling units have no kitchens and in which there is a central dining
facility. While these facilities may have some nursing care they are
not usually considered intermediate care facilities—a term set up by
the federal government for facilities serving persons that require
more than room and board and that require some medical services
(some degree of nursing home care), but not the full range. Intermediate care facilities have some nursing staff (at least a licensed practical nurse or the equivalent) on duty full time during the day shift;
these facilities qualify for Medicaid while most congregate facilities,
serving ambulatory elderly who can get to the dining room, do not
qualify.[16]

Lawton in one statement defines congregate housing as any
housing that offers something beyond the basic shelter. In this book,
Planning and Managing Housing for the Elderly, he points out that the
1970 Housing and Urban Development Act saw congregate housing in
terms of "need for services in addition to mere housing—services
short of medical care, which if provided, would forestall transfer to
an institution." He goes on to say that "one important part of the defi-

nition of congregate housing is the provision of personal services— assistance in the tasks necessary to housekeeping." These tasks are sharply distinguished from nursing care and are presumed to be appropriately performed by relatively untrained housekeepers or personal aides. People impaired enough to need nursing care are explicitly excluded from the congregate care facility.

Lawton feels this conception implies that there is a continuum of full independence, personal care, and nursing care. He challenges this concept, saying that "research has shown us that food preparation, eating, grooming, and housekeeping are skills that are maintained by older people up until the time when gross physical or mental infirmity intrudes. Therefore, it is difficult to imagine these highly personal, in-dwelling-unit services being required by anyone who does not also require some medical services that go beyond the usual doctor's-office care."[17] He thus adds that his version of the continuum of care would be full independence, on-site services, and personal and nursing services.

Lawton warns against providing expensive services if a large group of the residents do not need them. Some experts even debate whether "congregate" should mean dining facilities;[18] Senator Harrison Williams, Jr. says the 1970 congregate provision is restrictive as it is almost solely concerned with provision for group dining facilities.[19] However, to us, this criterion is a necessary component.

Lawton in his study of public housing tenants did find that many wanted, in order to feel secure, a number of services in the housing, including medical services, housekeeping, and meals, even though many would not make much use of these services. Lawton does mention that many elderly, lacking transportation, have trouble connecting up with community services. He says that "locating some of these resources on the site may prove a link for some people equivalent to the link that transportation provides for others. Thus meals, activities, and a medical clinic on the site allow fairly well-functioning people easier access to basic necessities."[20] Carp, in her restudy of Victoria Plaza public housing in San Antonio, Texas, found that eight years after her original study, there was a dramatic increase in the proportion of residents who desired a food service; 79 percent now had the desire.

This finding would fit in with her statement that "facilities designed to meet the needs of applicants are soon outgrown as the first tenants age and the age structure of the tenant group skews upward. This has proved true in both retirement communities for the relatively affluent and in public housing for the elderly."[21]

To avoid the expense of unneeded services in the first years of the development, as mentioned by Lawton, Carp puts forth the idea of an "add-on" architectural design and program planning, with expansion features possibly being health care, food, housecleaning, and personal hygiene services.

The likelihood that such a facility with such personal services is needed, whether originally planned as such, Thompson and others would advocate, or "added on" to a present elderly apartment project, is agreed on by most experts.[22]

Senator Williams gives the warning that "the clear but largely unnoticed emergency in public housing should receive early, cooperative attention by the Department of Housing and Urban Development and the U.S. Administration on Aging. Why should we wait for large-scale transfers from public housing to nursing homes or hospitals? Why should we fail once again to take preventive measures rather than give illness and helplessness a head start?"[23]

Donahue has made an estimate that more than 3 million elderly in this country can be considered to need assisted living, and that 2.4 million of them are candidates for residential congregate housing with services.[24] Mary Adelaide Mendelson in Tender, Loving Greed makes the more modest estimate that 200,000 to 300,000 elderly would choose to relocate in congregate housing every year.[25]

Many of these recruits would be people who would otherwise have to go to nursing homes. In fact, most experts talk of congregate housing in terms of it being a substitute for nursing homes. Studies of nursing home populations, such as those by Robert Morris and Matilda Riley, have found that a third to a half of those in a nursing home might be able to use alternative less intensive care facilities if such existed. Morris points out that between 250,000 and 300,000 people are annually assigned to costly institutions for reasons other than medical needs.[26] The U.S. General Accounting Office, after studying 378 patients in Michigan's nursing homes, concluded that 80 percent did not need to be there as they did not require skilled nursing care.[27] The New York State Controller's Office found 53 to 61 percent of the patients in nursing homes in New York City did not need to be in a home. The Krause Minneapolis area study of nursing homes gave the figure as 30 to 40 percent.[28]

Evaluating the needs of tenants among her surveyed public housing authorities, Donahue reports that, of those found to be impaired persons who were judged to require additional assistance, only 20 percent were judged to require a medical care facility such as a nursing home, while 80 percent were felt to benefit from a congregate housing facility.[29]

Most writers on the nursing home consider it an institutional setting that deprives the person of his or her freedom or autonomy or privacy. Kurt Reichert calls the nursing home a place for "premature functional death" and blames the shortening of the lifespan partly on the institutional process itself:

It may be assumed that all candidates for long term care, i.e., all those whose functional capacity is severely restricted as a result of physical or social trauma, chronic disease or aging constitute the population at risk of premature functional death, substantially caused by the total impact of the long term care processes themselves.[30]

In comparison, congregate housing may be said to be, first, a means to lengthen the person's stay in the community in a semiindependent environment. Second, it is certainly a cheaper housing arrangement than a nursing home, which ranges in cost from a low of $300 a month per patient to the more likely cost of $700 or $800 a month. The director of the Maryland State Office on Aging recommended HUD support of experimental sheltered housing, with a subsidy of $2,400 per year, or $200 a month. He said that "this sum is peanuts compared to the billions of dollars being invested in unnecessary institutionalization."[31] Susan Jacoby reports that in 1973 between $5 billion and $7 billion was spent on U.S. nursing homes.[32] However, unlike the residents of congregate housing, over two-thirds of the nursing home residents do not pay any of their living arrangement bill. Elaine Brody, cataloguing the flow of federal funds into subsidization of nursing homes, through such programs as Medicaid, Medicare, the Hill-Burton program, the Kerr-Mills program, and even the 1959 Housing Act, shows how the individual's bills are eligible for reimbursement, and therefore how residents of nursing homes have become main recipients of government aid.[33] Congregate housing residents are less likely to benefit, though some public housing is now becoming congregate housing, and Section 8 funds can be used for congregate housing.

A basic reason, however, why nursing homes will still continue to be used for the impaired elderly who do not need them is that the alternative of congregate housing does not exist. Lawton says the number of congregate housing units is "miniscule." One research group, trying to estimate the number, finally came to the conclusion that there were under 400 congregate housing developments in 1974.[34] In some cases, apartment developments have congregate wings or partly qualify for congregate status as they serve one meal a day and have a number of services and facilities, such as Satellite Central in Oakland. In other cities, as one housing expert reports, "the need for congregate housing has been recognized for the past several years. On numerous occasions the city social service department has had to place tenants in nursing homes because there is no facility in our community that gives the adequate supportive services for everyday activities of living that would enable them to remain independent."[35] The director of the Manchester, New Hampshire, housing authority reports:

Of 12,000 elderly people in the city, we now house 1,185.
We have an additional 853 on our waiting list, and I am
certain there are numerous others who would apply but believe that the waiting period is so long that it would be use-
less to do so. We have in our projects at least 50 persons
that probably should, now or in the near future, move into
congregate housing. We estimate that approximately 25
persons, per annum, move from our program into nursing
homes. Even the nursing homes have waiting lists, and
cost, at $500 per month, is a major factor. Unless the
elderly applicant has assets, he or she is not even considered for a bed.[36]

In New York City, according to Matthew Tayback, there were
in 1975 no congregate housing units in public housing in the metropolitan area.[37] In general, we know that although the 1970 Housing Act
allowed public housing authorities to develop congregate housing,
very few did. In 1975 some 400 housing authorities did operate on
some 700 sites a hot meal program under the nutrition program of
the AOA.[38]

Of the elderly units built under the Section 202/236 program,
a number are congregate. One source reports over 60 percent of the
202 projects in 1972 had dining rooms.[39]

One can thus see why the total estimate of congregate housing
is 400 projects. In some areas, ironically, there is a shortage of
both the congregate housing arrangement that would allow elderly a
semiindependent life style, and the nursing home. As the Richmond,
Virginia, housing authority director reports: "the scarcity of nursing
home facilities is another obstacle to local housing authorities. Without them, the low-rent housing development for the elderly itself
may soon become a nursing home. In Richmond, all nursing home
beds are filled and a waiting list exists."[40] This again points to the
need for congregate housing. This type of situation is especially
evident in rural areas.

Many congregate facilities have waiting lists. Almost a third
of our 294 managers of subsidized elderly housing in Canada (both
apartment and congregate housing) reported a severe shortage of
congregate housing in their area; 60 percent said there was a severe
or moderate shortage while 40 percent said there was some or no
shortage. Managers of housing in metropolitan areas were less likely
to see a severe shortage compared to managers in small towns or
other urban areas.

However, some congregate developments have not been completely full, especially in their first year. Experts attribute this to
the cost. In the many cases where services are not subsidized or

provided for by the community, and the residents are not on rent supplement (Section 236 housing) or the project does not have leased public housing tenants, the rents are, by necessity, higher than for the conventional apartment. Many elderly, while desiring the services, cannot pay these rents. Medicaid will not cover the bill as it will for the nursing home care.

Furthermore, in some areas, most elderly and their relatives are unaware of this alternative, if it does exist, and thus still turn to the nursing home. In a few cases known to us, the fact that the congregate development was in an outlying urban fringe area or, on the other hand, in a deteriorated crime-ridden inner city area, meant many elderly potential residents rejected it.

Most congregate projects do turn out successful. However, at present the demand is higher for apartments. In our Canadian study, the managers, at least those in metropolitan areas and major urban areas, were much more likely to see a severe shortage of apartments than congregate units (37 percent of the managers in metropolitan areas and 62 percent of those in major urban areas). Waiting lists for elderly housing are extremely long at most housing authorities; many die before they ever get these low-cost units.

Of course if elderly do get in these apartments they are likely to stay until they die, and that is why a congregate wing is needed. The head of the large public housing program in the province of Ontario, has pointed out that from his experience "with existing senior citizen projects, there is every indication that tenants will stay in these self-contained units until death or severe disability occurs."[41]

Lawton, describing the Philadelphia Geriatric Center elderly congregate housing project, built under Section 236, says:

Those houses, as one would imagine, have been totally 100 per cent occupied during the three or four years that they have been in existence now. The waiting list is tremendous for that housing, and my colleague, Mrs. Elaine Brody, who evaluated the impact of such housing, has some recent information suggesting that nobody has moved out of that housing for any reason other than for health reasons, and that the experience with the death rate has been lower among the people who have lived in this housing than in a couple of other comparison groups that she has worked with.[42]

This evidence on lowering the death rate of a group with a particular health status by providing congregate housing was also indicated by our research.

This all relates to the health of the congregate housing residents. All the above discussion indicates such housing is for the impaired person who needs supportive services. Data indicate congregate housing is indeed serving such a population, and a sicker population than in specially designed apartment complexes. Of our randomly picked sample of Canadian elderly living in congregate housing or congregate-apartment developments, 29 percent said they had a "moderately" or "seriously limited" physical ability, with only 7 percent saying "seriously limited." Over 70 percent had only "slightly limited" ability or "no incapacity." Interviewers, in their assessment of these elderly, agreed that about 7 percent were "obviously ill or infirm" and they thought another third were "somewhat infirm." Since almost half the elderly in the congregate housing were aged 80 or over compared to only 10 percent of elderly in apartment complexes, this is not surprising. In our separate survey of managers, a third of the managers of congregate developments responded that a fourth or more of their residents had "seriously limited physical ability"; in fact, 15 percent of these managers indicated half or more of their residents had "seriously limited physical ability." Thus, in some congregate complexes, the residents were almost the equivalent of nursing home patients, except they were probably more likely to be ambulatory. In almost a fifth of these congregate developments, ten or more people had died in the last year; in 38 percent, six or more had died.

Since there have been few studies of U.S. congregate housing, we do not have comparable data at the present time. Lawton tells us the death rate has been low in the Philadelphia Geriatric Center congregate housing. In my own U.S. case studies, I have encountered developments where nearly a third of the residents use walking aids or wheelchairs; I have observed others where very few do. In one, outside Minneapolis, many elderly were senile or had other mental problems. In two Ohio projects, one in Toledo and one in Columbus, one-third of the residents were ex-mental hospital patients, as the state contracted for these projects to take elderly patients who had no psychosis and who they felt did not need hospitalization. [43] At the other end of the continuum, in a Vancouver mixed congregate and apartment development, only one person was seriously incapacitated. Most developments use tests on physical and mental capacities and doctors' reports to guide them in selection. For example, the Maryland State Office on Aging, in their guidelines on sheltered housing, say "each prospective tenant must have a physical examination and a letter from a physician designated by the tenant selection committee saying the individual meets the required minimum standard for sheltered housing and is not in immediate need of daily nursing care." [44]

Lawton suggests the management also ask questions on degree of hospitalization in the last five years, sicknesses in the home, and use of glasses, hearing aid, cane, crutches, or wheelchair or walker. [45]

Thompson suggests assessing a person's level of function and degree of competence by such guides as the physical self-maintenance scale developed by the Philadelphia Geriatric Center, to measure a person's capacity for self-care, and the instrumental-activities-of-daily-living scale, also developed at the center, which measures the capacity of an elderly person for continued living in the community. A third scale, the index of independence in activities in daily living, measures the relationship of functional capacity to the accomplishment of daily activities. It provides a means to evaluate functional independence or dependence in six categories: bathing, dressing, toilet performance, eating, continence, and transferring from a prone to an upright position and back again.[46] In some categories, such as toilet performance and continence, the person needs to be completely independent to be in congregate housing, while for transferring positions, if he can get up with use of supports this may be enough; and in dressing, eating, and bathing, if he or she needs some help but not total help, then he or she may fit congregate housing.

Psychological testing is also possible but results may be more difficult to assess, as Lawton points out, and the testing may create anxiety.[47] Medical history and interviews with an applicant and relatives may give clues as to the extent of the problem. Most congregate housing developments accept applicants with minor memory loss or minor degree of delusions but try to screen out those with major psychotic problems, depressions, major delusions, or suicidal thoughts. In general they find they cannot handle those with major antisocial tendencies.

In our Canadian survey, a fifth of the managers of congregate developments, but only 7 percent of managers of mixed developments and only 3 percent of managers of apartment developments, said they would take applicants with seriously limited physical ability. Over a third of the managers of all these housing types would take applicants with moderately limited ability. A fifth of the apartment managers, but few congregate or mixed housing managers, would ask those with moderately limited ability to leave; over three-fourths of all groups would ask residents with seriously limited ability to leave.

Degree of Satisfaction in Specially Designated
Congregate and Apartment Housing

An indication that congregate living is a good solution for the impaired elderly and fills the initial objective of being supportive housing, may be the degree of satisfaction these elderly users have with the development. In our Canadian study almost two-thirds (61 percent) of all surveyed elderly were "very satisfied." Around 90 percent were either "satisfied" or "very satisfied." Apartment residents were proportionately as likely to be satisfied as congregate housing residents or those in mixed developments. However, older residents and those in poor health were slightly less satisfied than those younger and healthier residents. Obviously these users' original reason for coming to the development, such as rent benefits, inability to keep up maintenance of their own home, security and safety, need for help in cooking, shopping, or homemaking, or need for company, was met to a large degree by the development. The housing did provide to a satisfactory degree "an end to worries, concerns and responsibilities" that elderly so desire, as Hamovitch, Peterson, and Larson found in their study of retirement community movers. [48]

Since subjective evaluation by the elderly themselves may be overly positive, both because the elderly do not know of alternatives or because they want to please the interviewers, one must also use evaluation by other sources and use other measures. In our study the interviewers assessed the situation and they felt three-fourths of the users they interviewed were satisfied, with a slightly larger group in congregate housing than in apartments considered satisfied. The other fourth of the residents were assessed as having some criticism, or in a few cases, being dissatisfied with the development. The interviewers' assessment, case by case, of 303 elderly, was that two-thirds of these elderly were in housing suitable for them. When the interviewers felt a particular development that the elderly interviewee was in was not suitable, the most likely reason was that it was an environment lacking the social interaction the person needed (in 11 percent of the cases, usually apartment users); or that the development lacked needed nursing services (9 percent of these cases), or lacked transportation services or closeness to shopping that this person needed (8 percent). Other reasons were that the person needed homemaker or maid service (again in the case of apartment residents), needed meals on wheels or other food preparation service or had trouble living in group situations.

In the two-thirds of the cases where the interviewer felt the particular development was suitable for this particular elderly person, the most likely reason as to why it was suitable, given for almost a third of the residents, was that the resident had sufficient services and facilities supplied in the development. For another large group (23 percent), the reason was not that services and facilities were satisfactory but that the resident was independent, active, and capable of caring for himself, and thus could manage with the degree of services provided; or, for another 9 percent, that he or she had the services provided by spouse, family, or friends.

Carp verifies that this housing is a suitable environment for the elderly from findings of her study and restudy eight years later of el-

derly in public housing. She found a favorable impact or beneficial
effects from living in improved housing, not only as indicated from
indexes of life satisfaction, well-being, and desired life style, but
from the fact that there were lower death and institutionalization rates
for the public housing group studied than for the comparison group.
She reports, "not only has better housing increased the length of life;
it has also increased the quality of the extra years. The feasibility
of attaining societal goals for older citizens through the medium of
housing seems now to be well documented."[49] This can be verified
by other studies. Benefits following a move to an apartment house
built under the Section 202 program were reported by Donahue (some
of the residents were under rent supplement). Brody found the death
rate lower among people living in the Section 236 Philadelphia Geriatric Center development than for some other comparison groups.[50]
Associations between moving to better housing and various indexes
of well-being were also found, upon comparing movers and nonmovers,
by G. L. Bultena and V. Wood, and also by S. R. Sherman, and by
A. Lipman.[51] Looking at five different housing environments, and
validating across a time period, Lawton and J. Cohen found beneficial
effects of good housing.[52]

Whether elderly themselves find it beneficial and satisfactory,
as Lawton has pointed out, can be based on the number of users who
leave or want to leave the development; he found few in the Philadelphia Geriatric Center congregate development who had moved other
than for health reasons.[53] When asked, only 11 percent of our elderly
users wanted to move, and these were mainly people in apartments
who wanted to move due to lack of nursing services (half of those who
wanted to move) or to lack of meal services. Since, of those wanting
nursing services, only a very few were seriously ill and only one-
third moderately or seriously ill, congregate housing would have been
appropriate.

Waiting lists would be another objective indication of the positive
image a development has in meeting the need of the elderly. As already mentioned, most congregate housing has waiting lists, with a
number having a year or so waiting period; this is true even more for
apartment developments. About a third of the surveyed managers of
both types of housing felt there was a severe shortage in Canada of
such housing; about another fourth in each group felt there was a moderate shortage. Over a third of the managers of apartment complexes
and almost a half of the managers of congregate housing were interested in building additional housing for the elderly in Canada. In the
United States waiting lists for public housing for the elderly are very
long, often with more people on the list than total number of units.
The coordinator of New York City public housing reported that a total
of over 100,000 were on their waiting lists, including thousands of el-

TABLE 5.1

Degree to Which It Is Important to Reside in Same Neighborhood or City as Children, by Health Status

Health Status	Very Important	Somewhat Important	Not Very Important	No Answer	Total
Seriously limited ability					
Number	4	5	0	1	10
Percent	40.0	50.0	0	10.0	100
Moderately limited ability					
Number	11	15	7	1	34
Percent	32.4	44.1	20.6	2.9	100
Slightly limited ability					
Number	36	27	22	1	86
Percent	41.9	31.3	25.6	1.2	100
No incapacity					
Number	38	32	21	1	92
Percent	41.3	34.9	22.7	1.1	100
Total					
Number	89	79	50	4	222
Percent	40.1	35.6	22.5	1.8	100

Note: These responses do not include the 81 persons (26.7 percent of the sample) who said they had no children and thus gave no answer.

Source: Canadian user survey.

derly. Many Section 202 and 236 elderly projects also have long waiting lists.[54] In many areas this is also true for congregate housing, but in some areas there are vacancies due to the high monthly charges or to the fact that they are life-care developments, demanding a down payment. This again indicates many elderly feel this is a suitable and satisfactory means of housing.

Besides indexes of general satisfaction or well-being, in our study we looked at reasons for this general satisfaction and reasons for dissatisfaction, as well as reasons for satisfaction in regard to specific aspects of the living arrangement, including satisfaction with staff, with location, and with privacy. Giving spontaneous open-ended responses, a fifth of these elderly said the reason for satisfaction was privacy (had their own bath, were not bothered) and feeling of independence in the development; these responses came mainly from apartment dwellers. Another fifth gave design features as reason for satisfaction and almost a fifth (18 percent) mentioned "friendly atmosphere"; it was "easy to make and/or meet friends here"; there were "people my own age." In fact on another question, 43 percent said they had made many friends in the development and another 40 percent said they had made some friends. About 40 percent visited friends in the development daily, although those in apartments were slightly less likely to do so than those in congregate housing. However, friendly interaction was common in both and obviously a cause for satisfaction.

Other causes for satisfaction, each mentioned by 5 to 12 percent of the group, were convenient location, adequate security in building (including buzzer), provision of health care and other services, good staff, good meals, good maintenance, and good selection of recreational activities. On a separate question, most of these elderly users indicated satisfaction that the staff treated them with respect but many were not satisfied with number of staff. Only 69 percent of apartment users were satisfied with the number, and only 64 percent of users in congregate and mixed developments. Proximity of children did not relate to satisfaction as most were not concerned whether their children lived nearby (see Table 5.1).

In summary, indicators show satisfaction with these elderly housing developments is high, and the reason is that the complexes meet a variety of needs of the elderly. Above all they allow them to lead an independent life while receiving supportive aids. In this setting the individuals are neither isolated nor for the most part subjected to the extreme institutional way of life found in most nursing homes.

NOTES

1. Testimony by Wilma Donahue, director, International Center for Social Gerontology, in Adequacy of Federal Response to Hous-

ing Needs of Older Americans, Hearings, U.S. Congress, Senate, Special Committee on Aging, 94th Cong., 1st sess., October 1975, pt. 13, p. 894.

2. Testimony by Abner Silverman, counselor to HUD, in Adequacy of Federal Response to Housing Needs of Older Americans, pt. 14, p. 986.

3. "Housing for the Elderly," HUD Challenge 2 (November 1971): 7; National Center for Housing Management, Housing for the Elderly: The On-Site Housing Manager's Resource Book (Washington, D.C.: National Center for Housing Management, 1974), chap. 2, p. 3.

4. Michael H. Salzman, "Foreclosed Building Redeemed Converted to Leased Housing for Elderly by Efforts, Ingenuity of Los Angeles Housing Authority," Journal of Housing 32 (July 1975): 327-29.

5. "A Study in Successful Satellite Housing," HUD Challenge 6 (May 1975): 5-6.

6. Testimony by M. Powell Lawton, director, behavioral research, Philadelphia Geriatric Center, in Adequacy of Federal Response to Housing Needs of Older Americans, pt. 14, p. 1010.

7. Silverman, in Adequacy of Federal Response to Housing Needs of Older Americans, p. 1987.

8. Robert Taggart, Low Income Housing: A Critique of Federal Aid (Baltimore: Johns Hopkins University Press, 1970), p. 65; Irving Welfeld, "That Housing Problem—the American vs. the European Experience," The Public Interest 27 (Spring 1972): 78-95.

9. Taggart, Low Income Housing, p. 167.

10. Silverman, in Adequacy of Federal Response to Housing Needs of Older Americans, p. 986.

11. Lawton, in Adequacy of Federal Response to Housing Needs of Older Americans, pt. 14, p. 1009.

12. Donahue, in Adequacy of Federal Response to Housing Needs of Older Americans, pp. 894-97.

13. Marie McGuire Thompson, "Congregate Housing for Older Adults: A Working Paper" (presented to U.S. Congress, Senate, Special Committee on Aging, 94th Cong., 1st sess., 1975), p. 1.

14. Donahue, in Adequacy of Federal Response to Housing Needs of Older Americans, p. 895.

15. Frances M. Carp, "Congregate Housing: Concept and Role" (paper presented at National Conference on Congregate Housing for Older People, Washington, D.C., November 11-12, 1975).

16. Barbara Manard, Cary Kart, and Dirk van Gils, Old-Age Institutions (Lexington, Mass.: D.C. Heath, 1974), p. 36. The classification "residential facility," by Manard, Kart, and van Gils does not qualify even though this is a facility that mainly has personal care staff. This is because the facility is classified in national data on

nursing homes as a type of nursing home. And, in their book, several states reporting on such facilities themselves considered them mininursing homes.

17. M. Powell Lawton, Planning and Managing Housing for the Elderly (New York: John Wiley and Sons, 1975), p. 308.

18. Lawton, in Adequacy of Federal Response to Housing Needs of Older Americans, pt. 14, p. 1010.

19. Remarks of Senator Harrison Williams, Jr., chairman, Senate Subcommittee on Housing the Elderly, in Adequacy of Federal Response to Housing Needs of Older Americans, pt. 14, pp. 1012-13, and at National Conference on Congregate Housing for Older People, Washington, D.C., November 11-12, 1975.

20. Lawton, Planning and Managing Housing for the Elderly, p. 308.

21. Carp, "Congregate Housing," p. 14.

22. Marie McGuire Thompson, Design of Housing for the Elderly (Washington, D.C.: National Association of Housing and Urban Redevelopment Officials, 1972), p. 9.

23. Senator Harrison Williams, Jr., "Critique of Existing Legislation on Congregate Housing" (paper presented at National Conference on Congregate Housing for Older People, Washington, D.C., November 11-12, 1975), p. 5.

24. Donahue, in Adequacy of Federal Response to Housing Needs of Older Americans, p. 898.

25. Mary Adelaide Mendelson, Tender, Loving Greed (New York: Alfred A. Knopf, 1974).

26. Robert Morris, "Alternative to Nursing Home Care: A Proposal" (presented to U.S. Congress, Senate, Special Committee on Aging, 92d Cong., 1st sess., October 1971); based on data from the 1969 Massachusetts Department of Public Health study.

27. Mendelson, Tender, Loving Greed, p. 41.

28. Ibid.

29. Donahue, in Adequacy of Federal Response to Housing Needs of Older Americans, p. 896.

30. Kurt Reichert, "Social Work Contributions to the Prevention of Premature Functional Death," in "Human Factors in Long-Term Health Care" (report prepared for institute on health and health care delivery given at National Conference in Social Welfare, San Francisco, May 1975.

31. Testimony by Matthew Tayback, director, Office of Aging, state of Maryland, in Adequacy of Federal Response to Housing Needs of Older Americans, pp. 927-28.

32. Susan Jacoby, "Waiting for the End: On Nursing Homes," New York Times Magazine, March 31, 1974, pp. 13-15.

33. Elaine Brody, "Long-Term Care: The Decision Making Process and Individual Assessment," in Human Factors in Long-Term Health Care" (report prepared for institute on health and health care delivery given at the National Conference on Social Welfare, San Francisco, May 1975), p. 27.

34. Lawton, in Adequacy of Federal Response to Housing Needs of Older Americans, p. 1011.

35. Donahue, in Adequacy of Federal Response to Housing Needs of Older Americans, p. 1895.

36. Testimony by Robert McCann, director, Manchester (New Hampshire) Housing Authority, in Adequacy of Federal Response to Housing Needs of Older Americans, pt. 13, p. 923.

37. Tayback, in Adequacy of Federal Response to Housing Needs of Older Americans, p. 927.

38. Silverman, in Adequacy of Federal Response to Housing Needs of Older Americans, pp. 1982-83.

39. Interview with an Abt Associates staff member trying to develop statistics on congregate projects, May 1975.

40. Excerpts from "Housing the Low Income Elderly," testimony by the Richmond Redevelopment and Housing Authority, in Adequacy of Federal Response to Housing Needs of Older Americans, pt. 14, p. 1019.

41. Remarks by R. Michael Warren, deputy minister of Housing, province of Ontario, reported in "Ontario Regional Workshop on Housing the Elderly; Comments on Housing the Elderly and Beyond Shelter: Proceedings," mimeographed (Ottawa: Canadian Council on Social Development and Ontario Welfare Council, October 1974), p. 9.

42. Lawton, in Adequacy of Federal Response to Housing Needs of Older Americans, pt. 14, p. 1014.

43. "Congregate Housing Developments in Toledo and Columbus, Ohio," in Adequacy of Federal Response to Housing Needs of Older Americans, pt. 13, pp. 972-75.

44. Tayback, in Adequacy of Federal Response to Housing Needs of Older Americans, p. 962.

45. Lawton, Planning and Managing Housing for the Elderly, p. 242.

46. Thompson, "Congregate Housing for Older Adults," p. 19.

47. Lawton, Planning and Managing Housing for the Elderly, p. 243.

48. M. B. Hamovitch, J. A. Peterson, and A. E. Larson, "Perceptions and Fulfillment of Housing Needs of an Aging Population" (paper presented at International Congress of Gerontology, Washington, D.C., August 26, 1969).

49. Carp, "Congregate Housing," pp. 3-4.

50. Lawton, in Adequacy of Federal Response to Housing Needs of Older Americans, pt. 14, p. 1014.

51. G. L. Bultena and V. Wood, "The American Retirement Community: Bane or Blessing," Journal of Gerontology 24 (1969): 209-17; A. Lipman, "Public Housing and Attitudinal Adjustment in Old Age: A Comparative Study," Journal of Geriatric Psychiatry 2 (1968): 88-101; S. R. Sherman, "Housing Environments for the Well Elderly: Scope and Impact," mimeographed (Albany: New York State Department of Mental Health, 1973).

52. M. P. Lawton and J. Cohen, "The Generality of Housing Impact on Older People," Journal of Gerontology 29 (1974): 194-204.

53. Lawton, in Adequacy of Federal Response to Housing Needs of Older Americans, pt. 14, p. 1014.

54. Interviews with personnel at San Francisco Bay area developments such as Satellite Homes and Our Lady development in Oakland and Minneapolis area developments.

6

SERVICES AND STAFFING
IN SPECIALLY DESIGNED
APARTMENTS AND CONGREGATE
HOUSING FOR THE ELDERLY

Provision of standard architecturally pleasing shelter for the elderly is not enough. This is only the shell in which a community of people in need reside. To make this housing a satisfactory environment in which the elderly can enjoy an independent or semiindependent life style, one must think beyond shelter. These elderly have come to this housing because they have special needs, as documented earlier. Many cannot stay in elderly developments, especially the impaired living in congregate housing, unless there are services, facilities, and staff to take care of their needs. As our interviewers found for a third of our surveyed elderly, the development proves suitable mainly for the reason that it provides "sufficient services and facilities to meet their needs."

Many experts are realizing this service and facility component is necessary. As the National Center for Housing Management, in its manual on elderly housing, says in discussing the role of management in providing social services:

> To provide shelter, well-maintained and financially sound, has been the traditional goal of management and consequently the basic role of housing managers. However, it has become increasingly clear with social change that managers have to assume responsibility to see that the social needs of their residents (the elderly are a special instance) are met.[1]

This group warns in its manual that "the housing manager must attempt to provide guidelines in meeting these needs, if for no other reason than the fact that the economic and physical well being of his housing development may be endangered by ignoring the social needs of the residents."[2]

What do services and staff do for the elderly? The director of the Newark housing authority nicely sums it up by saying:

> These programs are primarily designed to prevent unnec-
> essary institutionalization, to alleviate social isolation,
> to provide health, education, screening, diagnostic coun-
> seling, as well as to provide a program of balanced nutri-
> tion, and nutrition counseling, designed to meet the needs
> of older people; to provide program participants with the
> knowledge and ability to run their household efficiently,
> and with a minimum of exertion; and to provide group in-
> teraction, and a sense of community in a variety of rec-
> reational and social activities.[3]

This is a big bill but some developments do provide the variety of services that covers all these points.

At the National Conference on Congregate Housing, Carp[4] emphasized four services: food, health care, housecleaning, and personal hygiene; Thompson in her report covered these and social programs. Lawton,[5] in covering on-site services for the elderly in either apartments or congregate housing in his book, discusses an activity program, including film programs, local entertainment, discussion groups, parties, off-site visits, games, dancing, religious services, arts-crafts-hobbies, music, and a house newspaper. He also emphasizes medical programs including a physician's office, nursing services, an on-site medical clinic, and infirmary, a special care area. Under the congregate housing, he adds dining room-meal service, a snack bar, and midday snack lunch. He also covers housekeeping and transportation services.

Below we classify these services into a number of categories, based on our finding in our Canadian research reported in Beyond Shelter. Our catalog includes the services on various HUD lists. These include the guidelines to HUD area community service personnel, which list as tenant services, provided by housing management:[6] information and referral, sponsorship of recreational activities, support for tenant organizations, orientation for occupancy, and training for maintenance and security; and, as services obtained from community agencies, health, education, employment, welfare, and recreation.

The HUD 1972 congregate housing guidelines include in the list of "additional services that may be offered by management or services obtained by management or needed from time to time: housekeeping assistance, assistance in bathing and delivery of food to individual apartment, clothes care—sewing and cleaning, laundry, assistance in minor exercise, personal care, counseling, friendly visiting, health services, recreational programs, educational programs and transportation."[7] Another part of the HUD guidelines lists types of services as health service, recreational and social services, special consumer services, emergency services, resident management services, and security services.

A report on supportive services prepared for the 1975 Congregate Housing Conference,[8] sponsored by the International Center for Social Gerontology, included as core supportive services: food service, housekeeping service, transportation/escort services, personal counseling and emotional support services, and social-recreational services, which included health and welfare counseling services (on SSI, Medicare, Medicaid, and Title XX of the Social Security Act), and information and referral services. Even later housing legislation, such as the 1974 Housing Act, has provision of services written into it, such as for Section 202 housing, presumably with HUD approval.

These HUD pronouncements indicate their increased willingness to see this service need. HUD has gone further and worked out a number of agreements on provision of services with other branches of the federal government, such as the U.S. Administration on Aging (AOA) and the U.S. Department of Transportation (DOT).

Yet some experts on housing the elderly complain that, first, HUD's efforts may be of a superficial nature, that is, vague agreements that are hard to realistically implement, and that, second, these other agencies are not coming through on the local and state level and providing the needed and often requested funding.[9] The local public housing authorities are in the bind. As Louis Danzig[10] points out, they must rely on outside service agencies to provide some basic services and these are extremely minimum. These agencies' commitment to provide a service to the elderly housing is often a short-term one, making long-run planning an uncertain business.

As Thompson told the Senate Special Committee on Aging's congregate housing hearings group:

> It is somewhat ironic that the very services that would
> support congregate public housing and assure its feasibil-
> ity all have been enacted by the Congress and appropriated
> for through HEW and the programs of AOA and Title XX
> of the Social Security Act. The problem, simply stated,
> is how to marry housing and the services programs into
> one housing-with-services program. Coordination at the
> Federal level, however well-meaning, will not bring
> either the planning or funding schedules together, nor is

there yet developed a way to assure services funding con-
sonant with the completion of the congregate housing project, to say nothing of long range commitments. Since
housing sponsors cannot commandeer the service elements,
and since congregate housing cannot succeed without them,
the program lagged.[11]

Many experts insist that HUD will have to take on some of this
service provision itself or see that certain HEW monies are used
exclusively to support the services component[12] in congregate housing and possibly elderly apartment developments. One cannot depend
on the generosity of other agencies since these agencies have their
own budget problems and have a large community constituency to
serve.

The past ineffectiveness of provision of services in subsidized
housing for the elderly, whether in the United States or Canada, indicates that some measures may be necessary. As Danzig says for
U.S. public housing, "the physical facilities provided by the public
housing program are quite adequate but are lacking in services."[13]
Donahue[14] found in her study that most of her surveyed public housing
projects had only a few services and many were not dependable in-
depth services. Our research shows the same lack of provision of
services by developments in our observed U.S. public housing and
in our 294 surveyed Canadian housing projects, as reported below.

Many experts, of course, feel the development, even a congregate housing complex, should not supply many of these services but
instead should use community resources. For example, the National
Center for Housing Management manual on elderly housing, addressing
itself mainly to apartment development managers, says, in its very
limited section on social services:

Although management, in most instances, does not have
the funds to provide direct social services, managers should
play the role of being the catalyst or connecting link in as-
suring that resident needs are matched with existing or
newly generated community resources.[15]

This issue of whether the community or development should provide the services is covered in a special section of the manual. In
congregate housing it is obvious that some services, such as meal
service and some type of housekeeping service, must be provided by
the development. That is why the crisis over funding and provision
of services centers around promotion of congregate housing, for as
Thompson[16] rightly says, congregate housing programs cannot succeed without a service component. Staffing must be provided in con-

gregate housing. Facilities, while more likely to be provided in congregate housing, are needed in apartment developments and in fact
are increasingly being recommended for such developments. Such
facilities as a communal room and even dining room and medical offices indeed are becoming a common feature in new elderly apartment
developments.

Since the issues centering around provision of each service,
facility, and type of staff are different, we move on now to discuss
each one separately.

SERVICES

Activities-Recreation Program

An activities-recreation program should be provided in both
elderly apartment and congregate developments. It is an unhappy sight
to see elderly listlessly sitting in a lobby or lounge of a development
or aimlessly wandering about the halls. This situation makes the elderly critical of the development and makes them lose their joy and
appreciation in being in a special facility.

Activities programs stimulate the elderly's interest and al-
leviate their loneliness. Activities programs meet the need to provide the elderly with a chance for creativity, for cultural and mental
stimulation, for meaningful activities to fill their day, for new hob-
bies and interests, and for physical exercise.

Social programs can help reverse the trend toward reduction
of social contacts and toward disengagement and estrangement from
society, which if allowed to continue can lead to lack of care about
basic needs such as grooming, eating, and medical problems.[17]
Activities provide chances for socialization and initiating new contacts;
activities can give people a feeling of belonging in the development,
of being integrated into a small friendly community. Community recreational programs can give these elderly a chance to get out into the
community and to avoid boredom and stagnation, especially in a small
development.

Most experts on housing the elderly now assume the development will have a varied and extensive activities program; HUD endorses
such.[18] Many managers see the need for this, even though they may
not actively pursue this goal or consider contacting community agencies, to provide programs, as a main part of their job, as is true
with many of our surveyed managers. Some managers also realize
that not having social and recreational services is a major problem
for their development, as 18 of our surveyed managers said. Many

elderly in these developments are demanding recreational programs; of our interviewed elderly, 19, or 6 percent, said their main reason for dissatisfaction with the development was that it needed more recreational services and facilities.

In providing an activities-recreation program, different developments go different ways; this may relate to a number of conditions. If the community has many social programs serving its elderly and the development is in a location accessible to these programs, the development may be able to make do with a limited activities program. For example, if a senior citizen center, an active library, or a church with an expansive social program are near the elderly housing development, then the development may not need an extensive program. In our discussion of alternative ways of providing services, we describe the advantages and disadvantages of using these community services. In our own study we found one problem was that elderly in these developments did not seem to be willing to go out and use community services. For example, of surveyed elderly saying a senior citizen center was available in their area, only 40 percent used the center and slightly over 40 percent attended church weekly. In fact, these elderly had participated more in community organizations before they came to the development than after they were there; a fourth had participated weekly in community organizations before they came to the development and now only 16 percent participated weekly.

Health status can influence the degree to which elderly participate and thus the degree to which one runs a recreation program in the development rather than have the residents go out for recreational activities. Our study showed elderly with health limitations were only half as likely as the well elderly to use the local senior citizen center. Health status also affects getting out an hour or more a day. More than two-thirds of those with no health problem got out one hour or more a day while less than a third with slight or moderate health problems did. None with serious health problems did.

Another factor influencing the degree to which the development needs to supply services relates to whether it is an apartment or congregate development. In an apartment development one can assume many residents are ambulatory and active enough to get to community services, although this is not true for all residents. In fact HUD indicates it is good to bring some recreational services to these residents.[19]

Congregate housing is more in need of recreational programs because, first, this housing is serving residents who are less independent and less likely to be completely ambulatory. Second, they are more likely to have programs because there is a manager and staff to stimulate such activities programs. And last, such a program is more likely because the congregate developments have facilities in which to hold such activities.

Unsubsidized developments for middle-class and upper-class elderly, whether congregate or apartment housing, or life-care projects, usually have an activity program, just as they usually have the staff and facilities for such. Retirement communities such as Leisure World of course highlight their recreational programs as attractions of the development.

Availability of federal, state, and local funding will also determine whether there is a recreational program in subsidized elderly developments. Some developments have been able to get appropriations under the Title III program of the AOA or under the predecessors of the Title XX section of the Social Security Act. In some cases there has been a spinoff recreational program as part of the meals-nutrition program under Title VII of the AOA. Some developments have had the local recreation and parks department run a program in their complex; this is true for a development under the Richmond (Virginia) Redevelopment and Housing Authority.[20]

Popular Types of Activities

In providing such a program it is useful to know what activities will be of interest to residents. Lawton[21] rightfully warns us that while there should be a variety of activities in a development, one should not be surprised if there is low use, with only a small core of perennial participants. Yet for this core group, availability of activities can make the difference between enjoyment and boredom in the development.

As for overall participation, not number of times a person participated, in our survey of 303 elderly users, 188 said they took part in some activity in the community room-recreation room; in total, they said they took part in some 432 activities; 97, or about a third, said they did not participate or they reported a community room was not available. Half said they used the room for special programs and a third said, for informal sitting; 28 percent said, for card games and another 10 percent said, for bingo and darts. A smaller number, under 25 persons, said they used the room for television viewing, for church group activities, piano and singsongs, special teas, movies, and birthday parties.

On another question, as to recreation available and used in or near the development, with most thinking of it being in the development, almost half named bingo and a similar-size group named cards and other table games; a half also named movies. Far less than a fifth named floor games, lawn games, and gardening. Many said these activities were not available and some said they were too strenuous for them to take part in (see Table 6.1).

TABLE 6.1

Use of Recreational Activities–Facilities in or Near the Development

Activity-Facility	Available and Used		Available and Do Not Use		Resident Says Not Available		No Answer		Total	
	Number	Per cent	Number	Per cent	Number	Per cent	Number	Per cent	Number	Per cent
Central community/recreation room	189	62.4	94	31.0	14	4.6	6	2.0	303	100
Senior citizen center	93	30.7	140	46.2	67	22.1	3	1.0	303	100
Bingo	142	46.9	134	44.2	25	8.3	2	0.7	303	100
Place for card and other table games	135	44.6	155	51.1	10	3.3	5	1.7	303	100
Place for floor games (shuffleboard)	38	12.5	84	27.7	179	59.1	2	0.7	303	100
Movie programs	135	44.6	71	23.4	95	31.3	2	0.7	303	100
Library reading room or mobile unit	130	42.9	94	31.1	78	25.7	1	0.3	303	100
Special garden plots	50	16.5	31	10.2	220	72.6	2	0.7	303	100
Golf/putting green	11	3.6	33	10.9	257	84.8	2	0.7	303	100

Source: Canadian user survey.

105

In the survey of 294 managers we asked a similar question. Given a more limited choice of answers, they said the room or some other development space was used most for table games (almost two-thirds said there was such use), while under half (42 percent) said television watching was a major activity in their community room; over a third (38 percent) said religious programs were a major activity; and a third said coffee hours (see Table 6.2).

What is popular will vary with different groups. For example, groups at different economic levels may have preferences relating to past activities. Middle-class elderly may be more interested in education activities, including lectures and discussion groups, and in certain sports such as golf. Ethnic groups may have different interests, such as in bocce ball, lawn bowling, or such.

More important, different age groups and health status groups may prefer different activities related to their degree of physical vigor. Some more impaired elderly want more passive and less strenuous activities; those somewhat confused or senile have trouble in participating in activities requiring a high degree of concentration or comprehension.[22] Those with vision or hearing problems may have difficulty with certain games. For example, elderly with hearing problems would not be interested in bingo while those with frailties may find bowling or golf too strenuous. Elderly that are somewhat senile may have a problem playing cards. These groups may enjoy movies, sing-alongs, or crafts such as using clay.

Movies

Movies were in fact a popular and frequent entertainment in many surveyed developments. Two-thirds of the questioned residents said films were shown in or near their development; almost half of the total group said they attended. In five congregate developments films were not available. Of the group that did not attend films when they were available (about a third of the users who had said films were available), the main reason was they "don't care for films," with two other major reasons being "physical handicap" and "other things to do." A few said, "too long to sit," "saw most of them," "poor selection." Others complained of poor equipment. Since a volunteer group or professional community person or tenant organization leader can easily take on both the job of ordering films and of showing them, and since the interest is high for both healthy and impaired elderly, as we found, every effort should be made to have the equipment and to have this activity.

Lawn Games and Floor Games

Lawn games and floor games seem to be less popular, both because they are more strenuous and, in the case of lawn games, require a good climate. In the manager survey only 15 developments
had a golf course and only eight developments lawn games. In the
user study the interviewed residents in only three developments said
lawn games or golf were available and then most said they did not use
them. The few that gave a reason said, "poor health," or, "don't
like it." As for floor games such as shuffleboard or carpet bowling,
less than half said they were available.

Bingo and Card Games

Bingo and card games are the undisputed popularity leaders in
recreational activities, not only from our studies but from others.
As for card games, we found they were especially popular with the
fairly healthy elderly and less so with those elderly with moderate
or serious physical disabilities, possibly because they could not concentrate to the degree needed. Bingo was popular with a wide cross
section of elderly; in the user survey almost half said the activity
existed in or near the development and they participated. Many of the
developments sponsored bingo games once or twice a month or more.
Interest of course varied among developments, with as many as 93
percent in one congregate development saying they participated and
over 75 percent in two other congregate developments. Actually those
in poorer health were slightly more likely to participate in this simple passive game. Residents living alone without children in the area
were more likely to participate, possibly because it was an easy activity to join in. Those who did not play bingo, when asked why they
did not, said it was because they did not like the game, or in a few
cases were in poor health. A few residents said they "don't like the
people," or "don't have time." A few users complained that at bingo
there were "too many people," it was "too long to sit," there was "no
loud noise allowed," or "not many play," and they "should have it
more often."
Since this is an activity that a tenant group or community volunteers can easily run, it should be encouraged. It enhances chances
for social contact with other elderly.

Gardening

Gardening is an example of a good outdoor activity. A number
of elderly like to work in some sort of garden plot and are proud to
produce a pleasant floral effect, as we found in a Dutch multilevel

TABLE 6.2

Availability of Recreational Activities-Facilities

Activity-Facility	Available in Development	Available in Community	Availability Not Specified	Not Available	No Answer	Total
Library room						
Number	83	81	3	113	14	294
Percent	28.2	27.6	1.0	38.4	4.8	100
Crafts, sewing room						
Number	71	34	0	174	15	294
Percent	24.1	11.6	0.0	59.2	5.1	100
Garden plots						
Number	92	13	0	175	14	294
Percent	31.3	4.4	0.0	59.5	4.8	100
Table games						
Number	174	0	0	97	23	294
Percent	59.1	0.0	0.0	33.1	7.8	100
Greenhouse						
Number	5	29	0	246	14	294
Percent	1.6	9.9	0.0	83.8	4.8	100
Bowling alley						
Number	3	100	1	175	15	294
Percent	1.0	34.0	0.3	59.6	5.1	100
Area for television						
Number	117	0	0	159	18	294
Percent	39.8	0.0	0.0	54.1	6.1	100
Religious service area						
Number	104	0	0	169	21	294
Percent	35.4	0.0	0.0	57.5	7.1	100
Coffee hour						
Number	67	0	0	191	36	294
Percent	22.8	0.0	0.0	65.0	12.2	100
Golf course						
Number	15	41	0	224	14	294
Percent	5.1	13.9	0.0	76.2	4.8	100
Card room						
Number	88	13	0	179	14	294
Percent	29.9	4.4	0.0	60.9	4.8	100
Auditorium						
Number	34	57	0	189	14	294
Percent	11.6	19.4	0.0	64.3	4.7	100
Mobile library visit						
Number	0	0	50	219	25	294
Percent	0.0	0.0	17.0	74.5	8.5	100
Group leadership						
Number	21	9	7	229	28	294
Percent	7.1	3.1	2.4	77.9	9.5	100
Social work counseling						
Number	16	97	20	130	31	294
Percent	5.4	33.1	6.7	44.3	10.5	100
Legal aid counseling						
Number	6	60	7	189	32	294
Percent	2.0	20.4	0.3	64.3	11.0	100
Food shopping service						
Number	1	46	6	217	24	294
Percent	0.4	15.6	2.0	73.8	8.3	100

Source: Canadian manager survey.

development (that we visited in Amsterdam in 1971). They are also proud to provide vegetables for their own kitchen. They can carry on a meaningful activity at the same time they get some physical exercise and fresh air. The elderly can watch the changing seasons through their garden.

In our Canadian research only a third of the 294 managers said garden plots were available for the elderly to work in. In our interviews with elderly residents we found that of the fourth who said garden plots were available, almost two-thirds used them. At the same time this data showed not all elderly want to garden when the chance is available; a third of those who had plots available to them said they did not use them. Their main reasons for not doing so were "poor health," they "don't like gardening," "there is a gardener," or, for four who did garden, the garden was "a problem when you go away," "too small," or there was "not enough room to plant."

Religious Services

Religious services were held someplace in the development in 39 percent of the 294 developments covered in the manager study. However, in the elderly user study, few residents (6 percent) mentioned participating in church group activities in the central community-recreation room; of course the developments run by religious orders, including several congregate developments, had separate chapels. However, since only 44 percent of all our users attended church at least once a week (and only a third of those in the nonreligious-order apartment developments), this would further indicate low use.

There is a division of opinion as to whether religious services and activities should be provided in developments. Lawton[23] points out permanent religious space is not permitted in U.S. federally aided buildings. He suggests it is desirable to encourage residents to participate in community religious institutions. However, one can expect that churches sponsoring elderly housing developments might want to hold activities in the development, especially in congregate housing with mainly impaired elderly. We were surprised that our surveyed Canadian managers in only 22 percent of the cases said churches had major contact with their residents and in 53 percent more cases said had fair contact; 26 percent said there was little contact. Contact was more likely in nonprofit developments but some contact also occurred in public housing developments. In small town developments major contact was slightly more likely. In general one must say, however, that church groups did not take as much interest in these elderly as one would hope.

Special Programs and Events

    Special programs and events would be one way community groups such as church groups could take part in the development's activity program. As mentioned, contact with churches was not always there, nor was contact with community services clubs, as in only 11 percent of these developments, according to the managers, was there major contact with service clubs, and in only 38 percent more cases fair contact. Major contact with service clubs was more likely in metropolitan area developments.

    At the same time, in some developments community groups did put on special events such as Thanksgiving and Christmas programs or other holiday events. In our studied Finnish-Canadian Home in Vancouver, the Finnish community at that time held Finnish holiday activities, including religious services, and Finnish touring events, in the home and then later in the new addition in nearby Burnaby. In Burwell, Nebraska, the congregate residents benefited from the ladies of the Methodist church bringing in homemade pies once a month for dinner and from the school and 4-H clubs providing programs.[24] In our observed Minneapolis area congregate development (Berkshire Home in Osseo) the local nearby school invited the residents to a special luncheon and special school program. Most developments have some groups and sometimes many groups that regularly, on a monthly basis or such, put on special events such as bingos, musicals parties, and even dinners. Sometimes the volunteer group is erratic in its assistance but sometimes it is a major source of help to management, reliably and consistently covering the special events program

    The professional community agencies such as the recreation and parks department or senior citizen center may also come in with special programs.[25] The development tenant association or development management such as recreation staff may also provide special events including birthday parties and the very popular sing-alongs. Elderly get an excitement out of a party just as all people do.

    In apartment developments there may be potluck dinners once a month or even once a week in the community room. If there is a young elderly group, which includes men and couples, dances may be another special event or even a regular weekly activity. If it is a middle-class, highly educated group the development might want to provide cultural and education events, discussion groups, art or music lectures, using outside volunteers or school district adult education staff. Even if only a few attend, it may be a stimulating creative activity for those, many of whom are not happy with simpler non-intellectual activities such as bingo, floor games, or even bridge, and prefer an educational learning experience or cultural experience. Those that said they "don't care" for bingo, cards, floor games, may here. A house newspaper may provide a creative experience for those residents who run it while at the same time it encourages a sense of gemeinschaft among residents.

More of our user sample (149 people out of 303) said they participated in the special programs in the community-recreation room than in any other activity; added to this were the small groups who said they participated in special teas, church group activities, piano and sing-alongs, and birthday parties.

Special events can and should include off-site tours and events. Many elderly residents who cannot get to these events on their own, due to physical limitations, fear of the problems involved in arranging such events, or simple inertia, will be excited about taking in events with an arranged group. While tickets may be obtained at reduced rates, the cost of the bus may be hard to cover for low-income tenants. Sometimes the complex can use its own minibus. We know many complexes that have succeeded in regularly running off-site tours and events for their elderly, including the Oakland Housing Authority, and the observed Minneapolis area developments. Trips can be to the local zoo, to a sports or musical event, to the local museum, to a holiday program, or shopping, or even a picnic.

Here, as with all other events, the residents, through their tenant association or other means, should be involved in deciding on the events and planning the trip. Attendance will be better, first, if tenants are involved in choosing what attractions they feel will be popular and, second, if management pushes the event through publicity and such.

Coffee Hours

Coffee hours also may need publicizing until tenants are fully aware of the regular time for them. They not only may attract residents because they provide morning or afternoon break for beverage and cookies, but because of their informality, which means the passive, the nonparticipants, and the poor in health will not feel threatened. In some settings social workers feel these coffee hours have provided the right atmosphere for the frail elderly to socialize more, without threat from the overactive elderly, and a chance to inform social workers of their problems.

An inexpensive and easily run activity, the coffee hours, were available in almost a fourth of Canadian developments covered in the manager survey. In the user survey the question was on a coffee "shop," and two-thirds of the residents who said such a coffee shop was available, used it; 37 percent of all users said such was available in the development. However, managers in the manager survey for the most part did not feel a coffee shop was needed if they did not presently have one.

Arts and Crafts Classes

Arts and crafts classes stimulate creativity and are found in a number of developments, especially congregate ones. Sometimes an adult education or parks and recreation staff person will come in to run it; in one case we know of this was paid for by AOA Title III funds and run for area residents. In some developments there is a special room for it; a fourth of the developments surveyed in our manager study had a crafts-sewing room.

Facilities for Recreational-Leisure Purposes

Libraries

A library is another facility many developments have that provides leisure time enjoyment to intellectually and creatively inclined residents, especially to those who like individual activities. It certainly seems that it is a facility, either in a separate room or as a corner of a lounge, that community groups can furnish.

In our manager survey, two-thirds said such a facility was available in their development and another 14 percent said it was near by; only a fifth of these developments did not have it so available.

About the same proportion of users in the user study (three-fourths) said the development had a library reading room available or near the development or was served by a mobile book unit; 60 percent of those who said such was available used it. Most who said it was not available were in three small towns, and one suburban and one downtown metropolitan area development. Residents under 75 seemed to use this facility more, probably because their sight and ability to comprehend was better. Those who did not use an available library advanced two main reasons: they "don't read much because of eye problems" and "use other sources." The few other comments mentioned included "no time for reading," "can't read," "read periodicals only." A few users complained that "books were poor and old," the library was "too small," and it needed "more periodicals." Our observed Finnish-Canadian Home in Vancouver, interestingly, had books in Finnish.

Television Areas

A television watching area is found in many developments and is useful to those elderly who do not have their own television set or enjoy watching with other people. Sometimes a part of the downstairs lounge or floor lounge is used for this activity. In our manager survey, it turns out that television watching was one main use of the community-recreation room. At the same time around 60 percent of the developments did not have a television watching area, and most of their managers did not feel there was a need for such. From the user study, the indications were that few residents watched television downstairs in the lounge as most had it in their own room. Besides this reason, others said they did not watch because it was "too noisy," they have "poor eyesight," they "don't like television," and "don't like the people who watch it." In congregate developments some confused and partly senile people did not watch because they could not comprehend the programs.

In talking about the central community room's use for television watching, we are assuming most developments have such a room. Data in the Canadian study show that over three-fourths of the 294 developments covered in the manager survey had them; almost all congregate complexes had them. Degree of use and type of use of course vary. One hopes the community-recreation room would get heavy use, but this is hardly always the case, sometimes due to management policies. In our manager study, only 39 percent reported this room was used regularly by all residents; in 35 percent of the developments it was used by only half or fewer of the residents and in 16 percent by only a few residents. Even sadder, 7 percent of these managers reported they used theirs mainly on special occasions such as teas and birthday parties; 2 percent said it was never used. The facility received far heavier use if it was in a congregate development rather than an apartment development. Interestingly enough, it was likely to receive heavier use in developments in which many residents had a physical incapacity.

Almost a third of the developments had floor or wing lounges and these were found to be more heavily used than the central community room. In half of the developments with floor or wing lounges all residents used them regularly, while in another 28 percent half or fewer did, and in 17 percent of these developments only a few residents used them.

Users themselves, in our survey of users in 19 developments, indicated they made heavier use of the community-recreation room than the managers of the 294 developments had estimated for all their elderly. Two-thirds of these surveyed elderly said they used this room when available. The third who did not use it or chose not to participate in the community-recreation room program gave as reasons, above all: "don't like the people," "poor health," "not interested, prefer to be alone," and "have own sitting room." A few said they "use floor lounges" or "do other things with family." Only one said, "discouraged by staff."

Community groups also made use of the community-recreation room in a third of the developments surveyed in the manager study.

And this room was identified by managers as one of the main areas where "people meet other residents to exchange a few words," as was asked in one question. Other popular areas mentioned were lobbies, halls, and, in a few developments, laundries or floor lounges.

Special Auditoriums and Card Rooms

In addition to a community-recreation room, special auditoriums and card rooms sometimes exist. As Lawton[26] points out, an auditorium in a large development can be useful in that it provides permanent, comfortable, well-placed seats for a number of activities, such as movies and musicals, sing-alongs, lectures, plays, and religious services. Few of our apartment developments, but a third of the congregate ones, had an auditorium.

Senior Citizen Centers

A senior citizen center is today a source of recreational activities, as well as a wide variety of educational programs, information and referral services, and a number of other services. These centers of course can vary greatly in programs and staffings. But many provide a place where the elderly can meet, feel at home, participate actively, or watch programs. These centers have greatly increased in numbers and in types of programs and staffing. This facility is now found in most communities. Some elderly complexes include this facility; this is true of Our Lady's Home in Oakland, California; Worley Terrace in Columbus, Ohio,[27] a public housing project; and many others. The New York City public housing authority has long provided space in a number of its developments for this and other services.[28]

First, having such a center in the development mixes community and development elderly. Second, it means the development will have a facility paid for and staffed by the community. Many experts strongly recommend trying to place such a center in the development, although there are disadvantages too, with the main one being that residents will resent outsiders and consider them intruders.

In our manager study, 10 percent said they had a senior citizen center in the development, with another 65 percent saying such a center was within five blocks. Small town-rural area developments were much less likely than large urban area ones to have a senior center in or near the development.

In the user survey, almost a third said a senior citizen center was available and they used it; however, another half said it was available and they did not use it; between a fourth and fifth of these elderly

said it was not available. Therefore in many cases where it was
available it was not used. The fact that many more did not use the
center than did use it is a sad comment, but relates to another finding on the low community participation of these elderly. Residents
of apartments were twice as likely to participate in senior citizen
centers as were residents of congregate housing, probably because
these apartment dwellers had less in the way of activities in their
development and because they were healthier and more independent
elderly who got out in the community more. Healthwise, for the
whole sample, twice as many with no incapacity or slightly limited
ability participated in the senior citizen center (if it was available)
as did residents with seriously or moderately limited ability. Of
those who did not participate when a center was available, a main
reason, surprisingly, was the "waiting list" for joining. Other reasons given were "don't like people there," "health too poor," "don't
enjoy the activities," "club not active enough," and "too far to get
to."

Tenant Associations, Boards, and Councils

Tenant associations, boards, and councils are a way to involve
residents in the development and make them feel it is their home,
where they help make the decisions. Through it they can help formu-
late and review development policies. They can help assess tenant
needs and be a vocal point through which tenants can make their needs
known. Regarding activity programs, residents themselves can best
decide which activities they want through a tenant group.

The resident council is an organization through which residents
can make a contribution to the running of the development so that instead of feeling everything is done for them, they feel they are helping in the operation, whether organizing recreational activities such
as off-site tours, parties, bingo games, and the like, or special services such as a buddy system or legal counseling, or a lending library;
or getting volunteers (or paid elderly) for development chores such as
manning the reception desk, cutting up vegetables in the kitchen, or
serving meals. In some developments they also run a newspaper.

A tenant council can establish committees, such as landscape,
social activities, maintenance, and food services-to-tenants committees, to help make development policy or to provide volunteers for
tasks in these areas. The council can help management make decisions on retention of tenants with behavior or health problems, or take
part in talks with such residents. They can alert the management to
such problems.

The tenant council is a structure through which resident complaints can be channeled and action taken. It is an organization through

which management policy can be explained to the tenants. Sometimes managers fear the organization; they feel it will become a center for complaints and a source for resistance to management policy, a sort of Gray Panthers organization. However, most experts[29] feel it is a needed service or structure in any elderly development that can serve many good functions and whose role as a troublemaker is exaggerated. They feel it creates group leadership that can be very useful in developing esprit de corps between management and users and avoiding the "we-they" orientation found in many institutional settings. For example, the food committee in a congregate development can cut down on the normal degree of criticism of meals in an institutional dining room.

The 1972 HUD congregate housing handbook gives the residents' council's role as "working closely with management on policy, aiding management in assessing tenant needs, acting as a communication channel between management and residents, initiating special projects and doing fund raising for them; and representing tenants in disputes with management."[30] In the 1974 HUD handbook, community service functions of the area office of HUD included "the development and maintenance of tenant organizations which participate in the management of low-income housing projects and to encourage management to work with residents' leadership to achieve better and more coordinated services for project tenants, to expand participation of residents in project management affairs and programs designed to open up better relations."[31]

Both Lawton and Thompson[32] support the creation of tenant councils, with Thompson pointing out that a democratically organized tenant group will relieve the manager of handling many details and will save the tenants and development money, and Lawton saying that the councils are the most satisfactory vehicle through which to channel resident complaints.

In our manager study, almost three-fourths of the 294 managers said they did not have a resident association. Both congregate and apartment developments were as likely to have such but participation was higher in the latter, with managers more likely to report "half or more of the residents participated" if it was an apartment complex. In two-thirds of the apartment developments having a tenant association managers reported high participation while in less than half of the congregate ones having a resident association did they report high participation. Metropolitan area developments were much more likely than small town developments to have a resident association.

As for tenant participation on the management board, only 5 percent of the developments in the manager study had a resident on this board and most had only one tenant on the board.

Since "tenant relations" was the third most mentioned "management problem" in our Canadian manager survey, with 30 development managers listing it, it may be that a resident association would be useful in more developments. A group might also be useful in decreasing the complaints made by 14 users in the user survey that there was need of change in management policies and need for better prepared staff to deal with residents' problems (open-ended answers given as reasons for dissatisfaction with the development).

Problems with tenant associations include, above all, the fact that many are inactive or run by a small clique. A manager needs to not only help the associations get started but also help them to keep going, giving what assistance he or the social work or recreation staff can, without seeming to run the organization.

Transportation Services

Many elderly have limited mobility. For example, a third of those surveyed in our Canadian congregate housing had difficulty getting places and another 10 percent said they did not go out; in the apartment developments a fourth had difficulty getting places and another 2 percent did not go out. A number of these elderly used canes, walkers, and even wheelchairs. Many no longer drive a car or can afford to own one; only 6 percent of our surveyed elderly in developments owned a car. Thus, in this automobile age, many are deprived of this normal type of locomotion.

Assistance is needed if these elderly are to overcome these barriers to an independent life and community participation. Means must be used to see that socialization with friends and relatives and in community organizations continues, for otherwise these elderly will become segregated and isolated in these developments to the point where they will feel they are in a locked institution.

Either this specially designed housing has to be close enough to community services and facilities so that these elderly can walk to these facilities or there must be transportation services available. Many developments are not in downtown locations or near shopping centers. The majority of the surveyed Canadian developments were not in downtown locations but in residential areas, isolated suburban locations, or fringe areas of small towns where it is too far for most elderly to walk to a service. In such cases transportation services, as Lawton points out, "can make all the difference in the world to the richness of experience of the aged tenant."[33] Transportation services make up for lack of accessibility of the development to services and facilities, such as medical clinics, shopping areas, senior citizen centers, churches, and libraries, as well as relatives and friends.

In our Canadian study we found that residents of outer area developments where special transportation services existed were more

satisfied with the accessibility of the development than was true in
the more frequent cases where the outer area developments did not
have any special transportation services. For example, an outer
area development had a nursing home adjacent to it that provided
transportation to the town center for residents of both developments;
another outer area development had its own bus. In all three cases,
more residents were satisfied with the accessibility of the development than were the residents of other outer area developments where
transportation was not supplied. However, we must report that even
in these cases outer area residents of congregate developments were
less likely to get out an hour or more daily than was true of downtown
residents of congregate housing. Downtown development residents
in all but one of the surveyed complexes had public bus service close
at hand, while outer area development residents complained of a
variety of problems with public buses in cases where a service existed
at all.

Experts, such as those at the 1971 White House Conference on
Aging, consider transportation a major need of the elderly. The elderly themselves see transportation services as one of the services
they most need, second only to medical services, as shown in one
large U.S. study.[34] In our Canadian study, lack of transportation
was a reason for dissatisfaction with the development. In the elderly
housing allowance experiment study (sponsored by HUD and conducted
by Abt Associates), the most important criterion of a good neighborhood, these surveyed elderly in eight cities said, was whether the neighborhood had good transportation.

A main way to meet this need is to have public transportation
stop near the development. In choosing a site, sponsors of elderly
housing should always consider how close the site is to major public
transportation lines. In the past many developments have been so
located. In some cases the management has tried, after the fact, to
correct a bad transportation system. They have tried to have the
local transit company reroute a bus route to cover their area, or
have the bus stop changed to be on the development's doorstep and
avoid long walks by their residents. In some cases they have pressured for a special bus to serve them. HUD is now also encouraging
local housing authorities and management of other HUD-assisted
housing to do this, that is,

> to establish and maintain communication with their local
> transit authority and to explore jointly with resident coun-
> cils, the following: reduced rates, at least during non-
> rush hours; rerouting of transit lines to better serve proj-
> ects for the elderly and handicapped; adjusting schedules
> to accommodate special needs; and obtaining special ser-
> vices and facilities.[35]

In many areas reduced bus fares for the elderly in nonrush hours already exist; where they do not, this is a complaint of the elderly.

Other problems our interviewed elderly residents had with the public transportation system, especially if they were in outer area developments, was that the bus stop was a long distance to walk to and in one case was dangerous in winter because one had to ascend an uphill icy sidewalk to get to it, and that there was no bus shelter. The elderly at the Powell River, British Columbia, development also complained the bus route did not allow them to get to the medical services they wanted. Other elderly complained of infrequent service. Many worry about trouble boarding the bus or having to stand or the unreliability of getting to a medical appointment on time or back to the development in time for a meal. At some U.S. inner city developments the elderly worry about mugging or robbery on the way to the bus stop or at the bus stop. To meet this security threat some developments have aides walk the residents to the bus stop. Some elderly fear harassment by youth while they are on the bus and try to avoid riding it at school leaving hours.

In a survey of 12 housing sites Lawton found most elderly reluctant to use public transportation; those who did use it said they did only one or two times a month.[36] We have found many middle class, accustomed in the past to using their own cars, unable to adapt to use of a public transit system.

Another solution to this transportation problem is supplying bus service. It can be supplied either by the development or by a community service; in the latter case the development residents may be only one group of many users. If the development is large the considerable expenditure of buying a minibus may be justified. One way to cut cost is to have the minibus serve all the elderly developments in a large housing authority, as is done in several cases. Another way is for the development to have a vehicle used for a number of different jobs and have the maintenance man or other staff use it one or more times a day to take groups of elderly to shopping areas, medical services, senior citizen centers, or such, as well as to take them to special events or on special tours. Another way to cheaply provide the service is to have a private driver with his own car, such as a college student or retired person, who does this for a short time each day; insurance problems and public utility regulations, however, make this difficult in some places.

Housing authorities may be able to get federal funding for such activities either through the Department of Transportation, Title XX of the Social Security Act (under its predecessor some authorities did), or possibly under Title III of the Older Americans Act, although in the latter case the aid would usually go to a community agency, which in turn would service the elderly in the housing development.

HUD in 1974 entered into an agreement with the Department of Transportation whereby DOT's objective was

> to coordinate mass transportation services for the elderly
> and handicapped with existing transportation services, to
> make capital grants and loans to private non-profit corporations and associations for the specific purpose of assisting them in meeting the special needs of elderly and handicapped persons for whom urban mass transportation services otherwise provided are unavailable, insufficient or
> inappropriate. [37]

HUD also advised local housing authorities and sponsors for the elderly of the provisions of Section 16(b)(2) of the Urban Mass Transportation Assistance Act of 1964, which provides funds through states to private, nonprofit corporations and associations, up to 80 percent of net project cost, for acquiring mass transit equipment and facilities for the elderly and handicapped. [38] There are strong indications that only a few public housing authorities have been able to utilize these provisions as of late 1975.

Title III of the Older Americans Act, which is the section setting up area offices on aging under state-federal auspices, was amended in 1974 (Section 309) to add transportation services, whereby the federal matching ratio in the federal-state formula is up to 75 percent for support of transportation services to meet the special needs of the elderly. While Title III is concerned with coordination and provision of services through an area aging agency that "will enable older persons to live in their homes and communities as long as possible," the deputy commissioner of the Administration on Aging in the Senate hearings on housing for the elderly in late 1975 said that "Title III can and should provide services to elderly residents of public housing and special housing for the elderly." [39] Any Section 202 housing can also be covered, in that an amendment to the Section 202 program description in the Housing Act of 1974 added that the Section 202 program will be supported by Title III of the Older Americans Act, and will include transportation services necessary to facilitate access to social services. [40] In many cases the area aging agency, under Title III, and not the housing authority itself, will provide transportation services to a variety of elderly in the community, including those in housing complexes for the elderly. For example, the Alameda County, California, Office on Aging has made transportation services one of its major interests and is providing taxi service to elderly in one community and working with another city to provide jitney bus service.

Many communities or counties are now providing some degree of transportation assistance to their elderly under one of these pro-

grams or others. In some towns, professional social service groups
such as the Red Cross may provide the service. Sometimes the service is to take the elderly to a specific facility, such as hosptial, and
that group has hired drivers and vehicles. In some communities,
these transportation services especially focus on the elderly housing
developments because of the concentration of elderly, while in other
communities the supplying agency feels these particular elderly are
already taken care of by the housing authority or by sponsors and
thus they should devote their agency resources and energy to isolated
elderly in private housing. In any case, if a community agency provides the service, the management must make a vigorous effort to
see that its residents are covered and that the service is run in a way
to meet these elderly's needs. There should be a dependable schedule
and this transportation service should take the elderly to a variety of
community facilities and services, such as shopping areas, medical
facilities, senior citizen centers, and libraries.

A frequent substitute for these types of paid transportation service is the volunteer transportation service; Donahue[41] found 80 percent of the public housing projects she surveyed had a volunteer transportation service. This can take several forms. It may be that a
community agency or a volunteer organization with the nonprofit development provides a squad of drivers and provides scheduled trips
for groups of residents to a variety of community facilities. It may
be that they instead take individual elderly to specific appointments
such as medical appointments, and, in fact, provide an escort service for impaired elderly. The volunteer drivers take elderly groups
on outings on special days.

In our Canadian survey of 294 managers about a fourth said
volunteer transportation was available, a smaller percentage than in
the abovementioned U.S. survey. It was more likely available in
nonprofit than in public housing. Of the fourth of the interviewed elderly in all 19 developments who said it was available, many pointed
out it was available in their development for specific purposes such
as volunteers taking church members to a specific church, or it was
available to get to a public transportation system; managers and elderly alike felt it was often undependable, or went the wrong places,
or was not of use to them. Donahue[42] also found some public housing
authorities considered this volunteer service no more than occasionally available. It was usually not provided by the project itself. Volunteers often do not show up in bad weather or during summer holiday periods or do not cover weekends.

A regular scheduled transportation service is not only needed
more in outer urban area and rural area developments, where facilities are distant and public transportation is lacking, than in downtown
areas, but it is more needed in apartment than in congregate develop-

ments. In many congregate developments there is less necessity to
go out of the development to the grocery store, as meals are provided,
or to medical services, as a clinic or nurse may be on the premises,
or to community recreational activities, as the development often
provides these services; others, such as religious services, are also
less likely to be found in an apartment development. Moreover, in
congregate housing more residents have difficulty getting around,
are using walking aids or are in wheelchairs, and are hard of hearing
or somewhat senile, all conditions militating against their going outside the development. These elderly need an escort service, an individualized transportation service to specific appointments such as
medical, or specific events such as a church Christmas party or bingo
game or theatrical event, as we observed in a Minneapolis area congregate development. These impaired elderly cannot go on their own
and be dropped off to independently shop or make a visit to a doctor
or dentist. To what degree a congregate development has this type
of marginally competent elderly versus independent elderly will vary
and have an influence on the type of transportation service needed.

However, some type is required because so few elderly drive,
and begging a ride from those elderly who do have a car may be a
solution that many find unsuitable, as we found in the outer area
Minneapolis development we observed. Relatives can help out but
they too are erratic and undependable, and the necessity of waiting
for their assistance cuts down on the elderly's feeling of independence.
Also, many elderly in housing developments do not have relatives in
that area at all; a third of our interviewed elderly had neither children
nor relatives in the area—44 percent had no children in the area.

In some areas, the elderly solve this by taking taxis; in one of
our Canadian developments, a group together ordered a taxi to go
shopping. However, many elderly cannot afford this financial cost.
It thus becomes the community's and the development's responsibility
to see that these elderly are not prevented from going to community
activities, visiting friends, using community services and facilities.
This means seeing that transportation services are provided and trying to put the development in a suitable location.

Medical Services

There is no clear-cut agreement as to what degree and what
type of medical assistance should be provided either in elderly apartment complexes or in congregate housing. Possibilities range all the
way from completely relying on residents using community services,
or having the community source periodically come to the development,
such as a public health nurse, to having a development medical clinic

staffed by nurses or a doctor and nurse, to inclusion of an infirmary.

Several experts point out that elderly apartment complexes are for well elderly. They also stress that congregate housing is not conceived of as a nursing care or health facility but is for semiindependent or slightly impaired elderly who are still ambulatory. Many sources do acknowledge that these[43] housing developments can serve populations with different health statuses and in some cases these sources have prescribed certain levels of medical staff and facilities for developments serving residents with certain levels of health problems. For example, Lawton[44] sees a development or wing giving a moderate (middle) level of service for marginally competent elderly, and thus having a medical office with daily clinic hours by the doctor and 24-hour telephone access to a nurse employed by the housing project or related to a community group. For the highest level of housing for the elderly, for relatively dependent tenants, Lawton is for daily doctor's and nurse's hours and an infirmary for short-term treatment or a special care area, for permanent semiinvalids, built on the site. In contrast, for the independent elderly needing what he calls bare minimum service he feels a weekly clinic with a doctor and more hours by a nurse is enough.

The director of the Columbus, Ohio, Metropolitan Housing Authority[45] suggests that the response to housing needs of senior citizens be established within the local housing authorities on three different levels of living arrangements, with level two, for semiindependent elderly, having a clinic, congregate meals, and other services, and level three, for elderly needing constant help (but not a nursing home), having a nursing staff available, with services provided as needed.

Other experts indicate they see need at least for congregate housing to have in-house medical services. For example, the 1972 HUD congregate housing guidelines say

> In-house medical services are desirable, with regular
> service hours, preferably 24-hour coverage through the
> use of para-medical personnel and health aides, with
> telephone access to a physician on call, and a back-up
> hospital relationship for medical crises or serious ill-
> ness. Clinic activities should include complete clinic activi-
> ties—such as eye, hearing examination, cancer detection
> and podiatry care on a fee-for-service basis. It would
> be useful to have a station wagon or other vehicle avail-
> able at all times for emergency use, and for providing
> transportation to residents as needed for referral care.
> As many of the employees as possible should become
> qualified in first-aid.[46]

These HUD congregate housing guidelines also suggest cooperative
arrangements with community health resources.

Many experts are much more likely to recommend use of community resources, although one must add that sometimes their focus
is mainly on apartment developments. For example, the state of
Maryland sheltered (congregate) housing guidelines,[47] while talking
of personal care services and assistance in one or more of six areas
of activities of daily living, and of 24-hour surveillance, suggest
community linkages for health support, and add that these linkages
should include transfer agreements with nearby general hospitals,
health clinics, nursing homes, and private physicians to insure adequate health care.

In the National Center for Housing Management's book Housing
for the Elderly,[48] little mention is made of medical services or
other services, but, to the slight degree that medical are mentioned,
they recommend managers use community resources.

The need for some type of medical assistance from some source
is definitely there, even in apartment developments. For example,
first, 12 percent of the residents in apartments interviewed in our
study said they had seriously or moderately limited physical ability,
rather than no incapacity or slightly limited ability; second, interviewers assessed that a third of these apartment respondents were
"somewhat infirm" or "obviously ill." In the congregate or mixed
developments the residents' health status was of course worse, with
29 percent saying they had seriously or moderately limited physical
ability, and 42 percent assessed by interviewers as "obviously ill"
or "somewhat infirm." These interviewers also assessed that the
development was not suitable for 26 persons (7 percent) because it
lacked nursing service.

Other researchers have found the same. Donahue in her survey of subsidized housing for the elderly estimated over 12 percent
of the tenants needed more assistance than was available.[49]

An example of the degree of need and types of medical problems
that residents of one apartment complex had was given by medical
externs of a Richmond, Virginia, hospital serving an elderly public
housing group's emergency needs. In five months these externs answered 75 calls for help in this 200-unit complex, of which 37 were
major. These major complaints[50] included chest pains, abdominal
pains, fainting episodes, injuries secondary to falls and cuts, skin
infections, improper ingestion of medications, and severe depression
and/or suicidal intent. Ten residents were advised to seek immediate
attention at the hospital for such difficulties as a head wound, possible stroke, seizures, vomiting blood, intractable migraine headache,
problems associated with diabetes, and severe infections and cellulitis.
Minor medical queries covered were about medications, blood pres-

sure readings, minor nosebleeds, insomnia, and such. This was all
in five months in an apartment development supposedly for well elderly.

One is not surprised, then, to learn that the elderly themselves
say that a major priority for them is nursing services. Of our surveyed users almost a third (29 percent) in congregate housing said
they needed nursing assistance; 15 percent in apartments said they
did. In some developments residents gave availability of health care
as a major reason why they were satisfied with the development; 21
persons gave this answer to an open-ended question. Some were dissatisfied with the development because of lack of medical services;
some also gave, as their reason for dissatisfaction with staff, lack
of nursing staff. Fifteen persons said they might have to move from
the development due to the lack of nursing services. Besides the
group having an immediate need, there was another group that worried that their future need would not be met. A number came to the
development to be near medical assistance. Many wanted the security
of knowing emergency medical aid was on hand; they especially worried about lack of help on the weekends or in the evenings. They mentioned cases of persons becoming sick or falling and breaking a hip
or ankle over the weekend and not being discovered until Monday
morning.

Lawton found the same for his 1971 sample of 2,000 public
housing tenants. [51] Two-thirds wanted some security-giving on-site
medical service, he reported, but not the full institutional coverage.
They wanted emergency service and a dispensary open certain hours,
staffed by a nurse and a doctor. Carp found, on restudying her elderly
public housing group after eight years, [52] that now almost a fourth (23
percent) of them wanted medical services in the building, but wanted
the services to be nonintrusive. This is likely because, as Thomspon
has pointed out, a number of elderly, especially well elderly, do not
want to be in a complex that looks like a place for the sick. In fact
this argument is given as one reason for not having on-site medical
services. On the other hand, they want the security. In fact the
major feature that attracts middle- and upper-class elderly to life-
care developments, according to the head of the development firm for
a number of West Coast ones, [53] is the security of having total medical and hospital care provided.

Congregate developments for middle class built under Section
231 also usually have some degree of nursing service, especially if
they have a nursing wing as many do. However, a number of congregate developments do use community services and assume they have
made careful enough selection of well tenants to avoid having anyone
with chronic or serious medical needs.

Apartment developments that do not serve meals, especially
subsidized projects, seldom have extensive on-site medical services,

though many now have a room for a medical clinic and an occasional
visiting nurse (in fact in Newark public housing developments for the
elderly, they had the room but no staff so they closed the room).[54]
Lawton[55] found that less than one-fourth of the public housing facilities he surveyed in 1971 had such an on-site staffed medical service;
he said when they did have one, it was a very minimal type, seldom
a dispensary or emergency service.

The apartment developments in our large manager study, in all
but two cases, had no nursing staff; none had a doctor on staff. A few
apartment managers (13) said they had home nursing on the site and
about the same number said the development gave medical checkups
on site. Three-fourths of the apartment managers said home nursing
was available from the community, but few said medical checkups
were. These both were more available for urban area developments
than for rural areas.

In summary, one can say there is a need in each development,
but developments, when they do meet this need, do it in different ways.

Cost, above all, may influence the development's decision on
means of provision. Ability to get funding may affect it. Many other
variables are involved, such as whether the complex is near medical
facilities. Its size and the health condition of the majority of the
residents will influence it. Admission and eviction or removal policy,
and existence of nursing home places, may also affect the decision.
While the whole issue is more pertinent in regard to congregate housing, where there are more impaired elderly, one also hears of apartment complex administrators not evicting impaired elderly, either
because there is no place to send them, whether congregate housing
or a nursing home, or they have not the disposition to move them out.
The crisis in public housing for the elderly is caused precisely by
this problem. When these administrators hold these elderly on,
medical services are needed. If, as one Ontario official said,[56] these
elderly are going to stay in an apartment till they die, then medical
help must be considered.

Unlike apartment housing, congregate housing has been designed
for the impaired but ambulatory elderly; they need some services but
are supposedly able to get to meals on their own, dress themselves,
and are continent. Yet, even with elaborate screening some will
eventually need more services, especially medical, and even become
nonambulatory. Their health in some cases will deteriorate while
they are in the development, yet they might not have serious enough
problems to need a nursing home.

How does one provide medical services for these elderly? As
Carp says, this highly controversial topic is in need of more study,
but let us explore it.

The way suggested by many experts is to use community resources, not on-site medical services. Some suggest the manager

take on the job of linking the development up to specific community health resources, and this of course is what is done in many cases, especially in apartment complexes. The linkage may be with a specific hospital, community health center, and/or visiting nurse service. One of our studied developments, at Powell River, British Columbia, had a specific arrangement with the local hospital. In New York City there is a special clinic serving the public housing complexes, the Queensbridge Health Maintenance Clinic.[57] Many developments work with a visiting public health service, though it may be that the nurse can see only those who qualify as poor and/or only the seriously ill. A visiting nurse often misses many cases, as development managers pointed out to us. The development may also have a pool of doctors who have agreed to pay house visits to development elderly.

The development may go further, as suggested by most experts, and have a 24-hour surveillance emergency tieup with one of these sources or with a nonmedical staff person who is on duty or lives in the development, such as the warden system in British elderly housing.[58] Some systems rely on the telephone and others on some type of alarm system or daily reporting system (as in an Amsterdam development we visited in July 1971), which can be activated from the elderly person's apartment.

A slightly higher level of medical service is in terms of having a medical office/clinic in the complex and having a doctor and nurse, or at least a nurse, man it for so many hours a week, with possibly the nurse there more hours; the visiting community nurse can be used this way. If it is a congregate development or large apartment development, it is suggested this office or dispensary be manned daily. It should be more than a diagnostic facility. One problem is to get a doctor who will do this. Many do not like to deal with geriatric patients, especially low-income elderly on Medicaid. The development may need to make an extensive search for such a doctor or one to make house visits.

The development may also convince teaching hospitals and medical schools to use the project as a training ground for doctors and nurses. For example, one Richmond, Virginia, public housing complex[59] has medical externs of a hospital on call in the building for emergencies. One problem here is the limited reliability of free student assistance and the continual changeover of personnel.

All these solutions call for extensive effort by the manager of the development to relate to the community health resources. It may be that he and the cooperating agency can get Title XX social security funds or other federal monies for this elderly service.

For congregate housing, especially a large one, a much better solution, though more costly, is having a nurse right on staff, either full time or part time. If one cannot afford an RN, then nurse's aides or LPNs may do, with reliance on a supervisory nurse on call in some community agency. The jobs done by LPNs should not be confused with those of personal care staff who, in congregate housing, might be hired to bathe, groom, and dress the elderly, help them write letters and even get exercise. Some sources feel this personal assistant can substitute for a nurse or LPN but we feel the personal care staff lacks the training to handle the kind of medical complaints given above.

These nurses or LPNs should not be required to deliver intensive care assistance as in a nursing home, as these elderly in congregate housing should not require this intensive level of care. In fact, some suggest that one caution is to keep away from licensing, as this might lead to staff requirements for the development that cause the costs of the development to be greatly increased. Most experts agree there is a difference between congregate housing and intermediate or nursing care. In most states elderly in congregate housing are not eligible for Medicaid. However, as congregate developments are new in many states, licensing problems may still develop. Definitions for licensing vary from state to state.

Another way to answer the need for occasional nursing assistance is to have a nursing home wing in the development and have staff from this wing service the congregate wing or congregate and apartment wings. Even when congregate and apartment wings are combined (but no nursing wing is included), there is more chance that one will have a nurse on staff than if it were only an apartment complex, we found. And, of course, the larger the development, the more likely that one can justify an on-site medical service.

Medical Facilities

Many elderly apartment complexes as well as congregate developments, as mentioned above, now include a medical office where either a visiting nurse and doctor can see patients or a staff nurse can treat them. This will often include an examining room. For example, most of Maryland's elderly developments include space for a health clinic, which is usually operated under contractual agreement by public or private agencies.[60]

The more luxurious congregate developments, including life-care developments, usually have an infirmary where a sick resident can be cared for during a short-term mild illness or even after he returns from the hospital. This requires a nursing staff. In our manager survey, over a third (38 percent) of the congregate developments and a half of the mixed developments had an infirmary, usually with one or two beds, though a third had three or more beds. Only 2 percent of the apartment complexes had an infirmary. Developments that had an infirmary were ones more likely to have a high proportion of residents with physical incapacities.

In conclusion, some type of medical service and medical facility is needed. The method of providing the service varies and depends on a number of variables, including cost, funding, number of residents with health problems, development location, and size and availability of dependable community services.

Social Work Counseling, Legal and Financial
Counseling, and Information and
Referral Assistance

Social work counseling and the associated workers are only available in a few developments in the United States or Canada but are services recommended for elderly developments, especially congregate complexes and all developments with many impaired elderly, by such sources as the 1972 HUD congregate housing guidelines and by Lawton in his book. [61] In our manager survey only 16 of the 294 developments, or 5 percent, said they had social work counseling; only six developments (2 percent) said they had legal aid counseling.

These services are often considered ones to be supplied by the community, sometimes with the manager as an intervening and initial counseling source. However, now many experts realize a development social worker can better cover the great variety of counseling and information and referral tasks involved, and they suggest that when it is a large development, especially if housing semiindependent elderly, a social worker be employed; the manager, busy with many other responsibilities, usually does not have the time and often lacks the necessary training (or even the inclination) to do the job.

The duties of the social worker relate to the social and psychological state of these residents. Let us remind the reader that many of the elderly came to the development because they were lonely and many were widows or widowers who had lost a spouse recently. A very large proportion had no children in the area. Thus in many cases past contacts had terminated. The change in role to that of retiree or widow has meant serious social and psychological adjustments for many of these people, with the move to the housing development causing more need for adjustment, not just in role but in life style and status.

For some of these elderly a process of disengagement[62] may have started that needs to be counteracted in this new housing environment. Efforts at increasing socialization must be encouraged. Deterioration of health may have caused both physical and psychological problems, even loss of memory, delusions, and confusion. Physical incapacity may have led to lack of mobility that causes social problems. These disabilities may also cause the elderly to neglect themselves, abuse or endanger themselves, or be exploited by others and be in need of protective services. Loss of a spouse may mean the elderly person must suddenly handle family matters never handled before, whether legal, financial, or personal. Methods of settling these matters and sources of financial assistance may be unknown to the elderly person in need.

A social worker can be of assistance in dealing with all these problems. At the simplest level she or he can act as an information and referral source. They make the elderly aware of agencies that might help them on whatever problems they have. Pointing out this information and referral need, the Richmond Redevelopment and Housing Authority has said of their elderly:

> Many old people who are eligible for financial assistance do not receive it. 6,700 elderly citizens in Richmond are eligible for financial assistance but only 2,200 are receiving old-age assistance, aid to the blind, or aid to the permanently or totally disabled. 5,600 elderly citizens are believed to be eligible for food stamps but are not receiving them. . . . These statistics have led city agencies who are concerned with the needs of elderly citizens to the conclusion that the range of programs supported by public and private funds is not known to the potential recipients.[63]

Besides information on financial assistance from various sources, elderly need information on the range of health services in the city, from medical clinic to visiting nurse services. They also need to be referred to homemaker services, to food preparation and delivery sources, to mental health assistance.

If no relative is present, the social worker may have to be a substitute source for consultation and decision making on these financial and health needs. He may, to an even greater degree, have to take on an advocacy role of first telling an elderly person, who is in need of help, about services. The social worker may have to contact the elderly person rather than wait for the person to come to him, and then, he must follow through to see that the elderly person actually makes the appointment, goes to the service, or such. In the case of physically immobile elderly he may have to see that an escort is provided; in the case of a somewhat confused person he may have to go with him, or see that an aide does, to fill out forms, answer questions, and provide documents. An example from our survey shows this:

Mrs. C.'s neighbors told the housing manager this apartment resident never seemed to have enough money for
food at the end of the month and borrowed bread and eggs
from them. The social worker found out from Mrs. C.
that she was eligible for SSI, due to her income. She had
thought her $1,000 nest egg of savings would make her in-
eligible. After convincing Mrs. C. it would not, the social worker had to drive Mrs. C. to the social security
office as she used a walking aid and could not get there on
her own. The social worker had to remind Mrs. C. to
bring her birth certificate; when the social worker got
there she found she had to answer some of the questions for
Mrs. C., who easily got confused and forgot.

During this trip the social worker noticed Mrs. C. had
trouble seeing. It turned out she had a cataract in her
right eye. Mrs. C. felt she should let it go, mainly because she didn't want the medical expense. The social
worker had to convince Mrs. C. that Medicare and, if
necessary, Medicaid, would cover most of these expenses.
Then doctor's appointments had to be arranged and Mrs.
C. driven to them. This was followed by a hospital stay
for the operation. The social worker had to arrange for
Mrs. C.'s apartment to be held while she was in the hospital. Then the social worker had to visit Mrs. C. in the
hospital. Last, after Mrs. C. returned home, the social
worker had to arrange for temporary homemaker help
while Mrs. C. was recovering.

Besides the advocacy role of getting residents to community
sources, the social worker should try to make every effort to get
them to participate in community activities, including special events.
She may have to publicize such events, arrange transportation, and
work with the community group concerned, whether a senior citizen
center, church, or such. The social worker needs to work on strength-
ening the link between these agencies and both the development and
the elderly population. The first job is to make the agencies aware
of the needs and problems of the elderly. Many agencies still have
stereotypes of the elderly; many, including medical groups,[64] do not
want to serve them or do not understand how to serve them. Doctors,
for example, may refuse to understand that the elderly patient is somewhat confused or has trouble remembering or lacks the physical mobility or strength to do some of the things the doctor suggests, whether
it be to take exercise or medication. The doctor may suggest special
diets that are hard for the elderly person to follow, especially in a
congregate housing development (even though the development kitchen

staff may work with special diets). The recreation personnel may not understand the kinds of programs impaired and also passive elderly best fit into. Drivers may not realize they need to help many aged board a bus or get off. The social worker's first job may be to educate the agencies and get them to see the need to provide services in a way useful to the elderly.

The social workers must work at getting the agencies to establish close ties with the development. As mentioned above, in some cases this results in establishing good special relationships between the development and certain agencies. This may mean the agency places staff in the development one day a week or more, as the Family Service Agency did in a Hamilton, Ontario, apartment complex; or has its staff come in for frequent visits, as was true for the West Oakland Medical Clinic in Oakland, California, which regularly held hours at an elderly development nearby; or places interns or field work students in the development; or gets their office or hospital personnel to give special attention to the elderly, as at a Powell River, British Columbia, development.

Establishing special relations with the community agencies may also mean sitting on their boards or taking part in community social work conferences as well as meeting those community professionals concerned with geriatrics. One needs a close relationship with the area council or office on aging, with the hope of getting some AOA Title III funds or sharing in their community use and doing likewise in regard to Title VII nutrition program funds and Title XX Social Security Act funds. All the programs have some provision for social services and information and referral assistance.

The social worker may also try to educate new development staff to the special needs of the elderly, to the subject of social gerontology, and to his role versus theirs and how they can all work as a team. In such inservice training the social worker will coordinate with the manager.

Besides information and referral, the social worker's direct services to the elderly can include helping the new resident fit into and conform to this group living. The social worker may be involved in introducing the elderly person to the development during his initial preresidence visit, giving him a tour and explanation of the development routine and regulations as well as services offered. The social worker may even do the interviewing of the elderly person and the person's family, obtaining data on the person's social and health history.

The social worker may also be called on by the development staff or the elderly themselves to deal with psychological problems they have while in the development. Some of these involve behavior that makes it hard for a particular elderly person to fit into the development or requires treatment by a more intensive care staff than the development has. It may be something as simple as the person not keeping up his unit, not fitting into the development routine (our interviewers assessed that 3 percent, or 10 of the 303 elderly, had difficulty living in a group situation). It may be a case of the person arguing with other residents. The social worker's job may include trying to break up cliques or assimilating newcomers into them. It may be mediating between rigid rules-minded administration and a tenant group who, for example, wants to use a lounge more.

The social worker may have to work with a person who withdraws from interaction with other residents and staff. The person may have developed a deep depression that has turned him from a sociable optimistic person to a person who wants to die, who is pessimistic, and slow in speech, body movements, and task performance. He may have lost appetite, and weight, have difficulty sleeping, and gives less attention to grooming and apartment appearance. Massive loss of memory, usually due to brain damage, may cause problems in congregate housing with remembering meal hours, how to play games such as bridge—a disruptive situation; for elderly in an apartment unit, there are problems that can be more serious such as remembering whether one has eaten, whether the stove is turned off, whether one's medication is taken. Confusion and disorientation can inhibit meaningful social relationships, nondisruptive participation in group recreational activities, or ability to dress and bathe. It may mean a person wanders out of a development, endangers himself in a traffic situation, and forgets where he came from.

Deterioration in both personal care and apartment or room care can stem from these conditions or simply from an unwillingness to any longer exert energy and effort, or, if physically incapacitated, from inability to keep up. Other behavior problems include suicidal ideas, delusions, hallucinations, and alcoholism.

A social worker can make the elderly person aware that he has these problems. If the problems are in the early stages, the social worker may be able, through casework, to have the elderly person correct the problem. He can talk it out with the person and try to introduce corrective measures. In dealing with the problems the social worker will work with the doctor, possibly a psychiatrist, and any nursing staff. The social worker may also help the development, especially a congregate development, to compensate for the problem. For example, the worker may see that staff remind the person of meal times, may have a housekeeper clean the person's room, and/or have a person aide or staff member help dress the elderly person or even take care of cases of occasional incontinency. He may see that there are protective services provided for the person who abuses himself, neglects himself, or is exploited. The social worker, while always trying first to work directly with the elderly person, in cases where the problem is advanced, such as loss of memory, and where the elderly person cannot correct it himself, may want to deal with the family as well. Sometimes a family refuses to face the fact that their parent has this problem; often they resent being told about it. In other cases the family was partially or largely responsible for the person coming to the development, and their decision was made because the problem already existed (even though they might not have told development staff about it). Our feeling is that family and development staff such as the social worker should frankly face the problem together; however, many developments feel they should not tell the family of the problem, until the point where they decide to evict the elderly person because his or her problem is so serious it can no longer be handled by the development.

If there is no immediate family, especially children, as in many cases, the social worker may have to deal with the problem himself or refer the elderly person for intensive psychiatric counseling or medical treatment.

The social worker's job may also be to prepare both the family and the elderly person for his or her eviction to another facility. No member of the staff likes this job, and there is considerable evidence that managers, both at apartment complexes and congregate housing, hold off on doing this as long as possible. This is one reason we have a crisis in public housing. One reason for holding off, as shown by testimony at the Senate congregate housing hearings,[65] is that there is no place to send these elderly, neither congregate housing nor enough high-standard nursing homes. Of our surveyed managers of apartment developments almost none asked a resident to leave if he had "slightly limited ability"; only a fifth, if he had "moderately limited ability"; and the rest, when he had "seriously limited ability," although five managers said "never" or when the person was "hospitalized." Managers of congregate developments were slightly more likely to keep residents, with a higher proportion saying they "never" asked a resident to move or only when the person was "hospitalized" (17 percent gave these answers).

However, when it is decided an elderly person must be moved because the development does not have the resources or services to meet his needs, the social work staff may be the ones asked to tell the person, often eliciting the help of the person's family, minister or priest, and doctor.

The social worker may also be the person to arrange hospital stays, see that the person's room or apartment is held while he is in the hospital (most developments will hold a paid room for so many weeks), and visit him in the hospital if time allows. This staff may also be responsible for trying to fit the person back into the development, including seeing that he gets temporary homemaker or house-keeping assistance.

A different type of counseling the social worker may do is in regard to financial matters, where the elderly person has not had experience in this area or, more likely, is confused and unable to handle such, and a family does not exist. Or it may be legal advice in case of an unsettled estate, sale of assets, or even assignment of guardianship; if children exist they can, of course, handle these.

Another job social work staff might do is help develop and keep active a tenant association. Staying in the background, the social worker may nevertheless see that the group meets, jobs are assigned, and tasks are accomplished. They will act as "enablers," whether for the monthly meeting, community outing, or tenant volunteer work. They may be the ones to recruit tenants for the development jobs or such community action programs as foster grandparents, hospital aides, and the like. Developing group leadership will be a part of this job.

If there is no recreational staff in the development, the social worker may be responsible both for contacting community recreational agencies and possibly running a limited program himself.

Social Contact Services

The social worker is also likely to be involved in setting up such contact services as a buddy system, friendly visiting, and telephone contact service; the latter two are often available in the community, serving elderly in private housing as well. These services assure contact with lonely and sickly elderly, usually once a day or at least weekly and in emergencies. These services can be an early warning system as to problems. Where the development has little or no staff the buddy system is considered an answer to emergency needs, a sort of 24-hour surveillance system. Even experts talk of it in this way.

The buddy system involves pairing residents, usually on the same floor, and having them maintain frequent contact with each other and see that assistance is provided to the other if necessary. In some developments well or competent residents are paired with the more sickly and less competent elderly. A staff member or the tenant organization is usually responsible for keeping the service going. This can be a problem, as, in our user survey, we found many systems were somewhat inoperative. Over a third of the managers in the survey of 294 developments said they had such a system. Surprisingly, the apartment developments were more likely to have a buddy system. In this user survey, use was concentrated in five out of the 19 included developments, but even here usually a third in the development used the service; in two other developments between 15 percent and a fifth used it; in four other developments a few did. When a buddy system did exist, the most common reason for elderly not using it was that they kept in touch with their own friends on an informal basis. Others said a buddy system was for singles whereas they lived with a spouse or friend. Some said the system did not work well because of lack of cooperation, or the service was used only when a resident was sick. In some developments a system was started but then let falter, and interest died down, especially when no emergency occurred over a number of months (see Table 6.3).

Friendly visiting is a service where volunteers visit elderly in the development; in some cases they visit just the elderly considered impaired or isolated; often this visiting is on a one-to-one basis with a volunteer taking responsibility for visiting one particular elderly person. The visitor provides companionship and checks on the person's health and on his or her needs, either filling them or making referral to proper sources. Of our surveyed managers, a third of these 294 reported this service existed in their development; double the proportion of congregate housing managers, compared to apartment complex managers, said such a service was available in their development.

In our user study we found use concentrated in four of the 19 developments; 14 percent of the 303 used such a service. The few who had comments said they "didn't use it" as, instead, had family visit them, they "did not need it," were "too busy" to have visits, "visits were only made to members of the sponsoring organization," or they "didn't like the people who run the service."

A telephone contact service has the same purpose as friendly visiting but the contact is made over the phone. Volunteers agree to call a particular elderly person each day or weekly and establish a relationship and continuous contact this way. They again are checking on the elderly person's health and needs. In our manager survey, only 17 percent said they had such a service available to their developments; congregate developments were slightly more likely to have it available. Only two of our users in the user study participated in such a service.

Meal Services

Meal service is a major feature of congregate housing, with congregate meaning housing with provision of three meals a day in most circles. Subsidized apartment developments for the elderly have traditionally not offered meals but this is now beginning to change, with some offering at least a noon meal. In our Canadian manager study only a few of the apartment developments offered hot meals even

TABLE 6.3

Availability of Social Contact Services

Service	Available	Not Available	No Answer	Total
Buddy system				
Number	102	165	27	294
Percent	34.7	56.1	9.2	100
Friendly visiting				
Number	88	174	32	294
Percent	29.9	59.2	10.9	100
Telephone contact				
Number	45	222	27	294
Percent	15.3	75.5	9.2	100
Volunteer transportation				
Number	66	204	24	294
Percent	22.4	69.4	8.2	100
Telephone in each unit				
Number	208	72	14	294
Percent	70.7	24.4	4.9	100

Source: Canadian manager survey.

once a day, but in some mixed congregate and apartment complexes
the apartment dwellers could take meals in the dining room either on
a permanent or temporary basis. In the United States in 1971 Lawton[66]
found that less than a fifth of the public housing projects he surveyed
had any meal services, and when provided, meal services were limited to one to five lunches per week. Since then the Title VII nutrition-
meals program of AOA has been introduced and as of the fall of 1975,
700 housing projects in 400 public housing authorities were using this
AOA meals program, according to HUD sources.[67]
    There are a number of issues centering around supplying a
meals services, whether one meal a day or three. Yet there are many
benefits from a meal service. First, it assures that the elderly person is getting nutritious food and is related to the body's ability to
resist infection, to withstand stress, and to avoid physical and mental
metabolic disorders, as Caroline van Mason points out. In a number
of cases elderly persons do not fix nutritionally sound meals because
they are not educated to preparing such, live alone, and do not want
to bother cooking full meals, or cannot afford to do so. Second, many

elderly have difficulty preparing meals (almost a fourth of our Canadian elderly did) or difficulty in going shopping (as a third of our respondents did). Thus provision of at least one hot meal a day can be very useful to many elderly. In fact if the service is not provided some may have to leave the development. A few of our surveyed elderly, when asked if they might have to leave, said yes, because they needed a meal service; some gave lack of meal service as a reason they were dissatisfied with the project. Researchers interviewing this elderly sample assessed that for nine persons the development was unsuitable because it lacked a meal service or an available meals-on-wheels program.

In a large sample of U.S. public housing tenants Lawton[68] surveyed, half said they desired an on-site meal service. Over three-fourths of the Victoria Plaza public housing residents restudied by Carp,[69] eight years after her original study, now desired a food service or some place to buy a meal.

Besides meal services being a preventive health measure, for many elderly these meal periods are beneficial as times for socializing. They are a communal experience. As a tenant in a Niagara Falls, New York, elderly project said:

> In our building, I see many people who show the subtle but constant evidence of physical decline. Perhaps often a form of malnutrition. Quick evaluation might conclude that proper food and diet regulation is all that is needed to correct the situation. I disagree.
>
> The depressing and sickening circumstances of day in and day out eating alone is the true deterioration factor. In my humble opinion a glass of milk and a biscuit consumed in the happy and loving companionship of others, could be a more healthful benefit than meals-on-wheels, where one must still eat alone, or the funded nutritional program . . . [at] two church locations.[70]

The dining room provides a social setting where once a day elderly persons who otherwise might be isolated have a chance to get together. It is a time when their daily health condition can be watched, where the elderly can be encouraged to take part in other activities, and where referral to needed agencies can occur. Meal periods can provide a sense of routine and a sense of purpose for the day for these retired persons. Eating as a group can be a great boost to morale for the person who feels he lacks a purpose or for whom the day is meaningless. A meal schedule establishes an atmosphere of normalcy for his day. Elderly on the AOA nutrition-meals program have made such statements as "I had nobody to talk to until I came to this nutri-

tion project, and now I have friends, where before I didn't, since all
my friends had died off." AOA officials themselves feel the social
benefits are considered an important dividend of the program.[71]

Meal Services for Apartment Dwellers

Since the expense of a kitchen has already been laid out for each
unit in an apartment development, it may be hard to justify a full
three-meal-a-day service if most of the tenants are competent elderly.
Luxury life-care developments, of course, usually have apartments
and are congregate, serving three meals a day. Developers of these
say women, always having had a kitchen, want one in their apartment.[72]
Most newer subsidized elderly apartment projects have included
some limited community kitchen facility and some of the older public
housing ones have used modernization money for converting space to
this use. Therefore the apartment projects are able to accommodate
some sort of meal project such as a community noon meal program.
Over 700 of the public housing projects are running an AOA Title VII
program[73] for that neighborhood, usually a noon meal five days a
week. This program pays for a good part of the meal cost; there is
a low charge to recipients but no means test, and no one can be
turned away. The program is designed "to meet the nutritional and
socialization needs of elderly who are felt to not eat adequately because they cannot afford to do so or lack knowledge and/or skills to
select and prepare nourishing and well-balanced meals or they have
limited mobility which may impair their capacity to shop and cook for
themselves or they have feelings of rejection and loneliness which ob-
literate the incentive to prepare and eat a meal alone."[74] Since up
to a fifth of the AOA nutrition-meals program funds can be used for
the supportive services that must be included, this AOA program is
a real help to any housing project.
There are, however, some problems in utilizing the program
even though there has been an agreement signed between HUD and
AOA over the use of the programs in elderly public housing projects.
First, some elderly public housing projects still lack a communal
room or dining room where the meal can be served. While under the
HUD modernization program the authority can use some of the funds
to provide such a room, and many do, some complain they should
not have to use their limited modernization money for this purpose.
Other authorities hate to commit themselves to a dining room when
they are not sure of a long-term commitment by AOA to provide these
meals. As Abner Silverman of HUD said:

One of the problems . . . is knowing in advance, before you
make a commitment to build, that you are going to have these

programs, and they will be funded, and that you are going to proceed with a finished package. Certainly it is more efficient to design a dining room at the start and not convert a space to a dining room later.[75]

A second problem is that, regardless of the agreement between HUD and AOA, in some areas, because there is a high demand for the nutrition program and competition for the limited funds, the local administering agency is pressured to use program sites other than public housing. Voluntary agencies, beset with financial problems and possibly underutilized, see this as a chance to improve their situation as agencies serving the elderly; under the program they even may get funds to upgrade their facilities to accommodate the program. Also, in some social service circles, elderly public housing tenants are looked on as being a privileged group already receiving assistance. A third problem is that, due to the past traditional role of the local housing authority (LHA) as mainly provider of housing, many agencies do not see them as having the ability to deliver social services, a part of the nutrition program.[76] A fourth reason why public housing projects are not preferred as nutrition program sites is that the program is aimed at the whole neighborhood, and the providers feel there may be restrictions on using public housing space, or at least neighborhood people may feel unwanted or even prefer not to come to a public housing meal site. In the 1975 Senate Special Committee on Aging hearings, it was reported that one Newark project got the community rooms and was all set for a meal program, but the funding sources did not come through and no program got started.[77] In some cases the public housing agency has not been interested in the program because of the omission of specific incentives for LHAs to serve the interest of the Title VII local administrative agencies, or because they think their job is mainly providing shelter, or they do not have a manager to develop the necessary negotiations with AOA's local agency.

If the elderly residents instead are asked to utilize this AOA nutrition-meals program at a nearby site, it has the advantage of getting them into the community and mixing with other elderly, but it has disadvantages, as one Niagara Falls elderly tenant leader pointed out at the Senate hearing:

The funded nutrition program posts a bulletin in lobby [of the project] every week, offering aid in a five-day noontime lunch service. The distance of the two church locations creates a task for those who are handicapped or find mobility difficult. Bad weather magnifies this condition. Transportation service that is offered is limited because

of sporadic schedule. The services are in every sense
too limited to be satisfying. [78]

One way to solve this and get residents to these community meals
services is to provide good transportation, say, through a development minibus. Better yet, maybe bring the community program to
the development. One can have community elderly and resident elderly sharing meals, but not having to go outside the development,
when one has a neighborhood senior citizen center or day care center
in the development, with AOA or another source as a sponsor of the
meal service.

This noon meal can be catered, or cooked in the development
kitchen. Many developments now find catering simpler and cheaper,
and it saves them the cost of building or converting to a full kitchen
facility. They still need a communal room or dining room, but there
can be a limited kitchen. Hospitals, schools, and private restaurants
have been utilized as caterers. For example, Burwell, Nebraska,
congregate housing uses a hospital as caterers. [79] Part of the service can be buffet to cut down on staff, although the disabled elderly
will then need help. The elderly themselves can be used to set up
the lunch and clear the table. In many places where the meal is
cooked on the premises, these elderly residents help prepare and
cook the food.

Some apartment developments meet this meal service problem
by having an elderly resident cook a meal for the other residents once
a week in her apartment. Some developments also have monthly or
even weekly potluck dinners.

Apartment developments may provide partial assistance on this
meal problem by providing a coffee bar, snack room, and/or small
grocery store. The coffee bar may be self-service for midmorning
or midafternoon snacks, such as coffee and Danish pastry or dough-
nuts; it may operate all day. Tenant association volunteers may staff
it to the degree needed. One life-care development provided a coffee
bar for awhile, and it was felt it gave tenants an alternative to getting
up for the breakfast routine and also gave them a place for informal
contact. Passive and frail elderly may find it a pleasant place to interact without the need to actively participate.

A snack bar-grill setup may serve a more complete breakfast
and lunch; it will need staffing. A small grocery store will mean residents do not need to go out for supplies in bad weather or when sickly
or disabled.

In the Canadian manager study the coffee room was available
in 14 percent of the apartment developments and 42 percent of the
congregate and mixed developments. Managers who did not have a
coffee room did not seem to feel it was needed. A third of the managers said they ran a coffee hour someplace in the development.

In the user study over a third of the residents said a coffee shop was available, and of this group almost two-thirds said they used it. Some reasons residents gave for not using it when it was available were, above all, "have snacks in my room," followed by "too expensive," "don't like the atmosphere," "go to restaurants."

A minigrocery-general store, here called "tuck" shop, was available in 63 percent of the developments. Grocery service from the community was available in a fifth of the developments. This is an easy service to arrange, and grocery stores should be located that will make such deliveries to development elderly. Many grocery stores will charge for this delivery.

A community service existing in many areas to help with the food preparation problem is the meals-on-wheels program whereby a hot meal is delivered to the elderly's apartment each noon. This community service is often provided by volunteer groups, with a hospital, school, or such preparing the meals, which are put in special containers to keep warm during delivery by volunteers. About a third of the 294 surveyed housing managers said the service was available from the community; 15 said it was available from the development. In the user study only four apartment dwellers out of the many saying they had difficulty cooking regularly used such a service. Some of the complaints against the service were that it was "too expensive," "not available on weekends," or the food was "not good" or "cold upon arrival."

Community homemaker services can also include cooking a noon meal or several meals. One-third of the developments in Canada has such a service available in their community.

Meals in Congregate Housing

In congregate housing it is assumed that three meals a day will be provided. Since these are mainly impaired elderly who often have difficulty cooking, the service is needed.

The AOA nutrition-meals program will usually not cover the need as it provides only one meal a day, usually at noon. However, the AOA meal program can be used to reduce the total cost of providing the service in a development. Cost is a major problem. This meal service is one of the major expenses of congregate developments. According to Van Mason,[80] in 1975 raw food costs at one large establishment for the elderly were $1.90 a day per person. In another they had to charge $1 for breakfast, $1.50 for lunch, and $1 for supper, to cover their cost of help, supplies, equipment, and raw food; raw food costs were 45 percent of the cost.

Thompson[81] gives food costs as a main reason why there has not been nationwide implementation of the congregate housing program

She and Lawton point out the inability of low-income elderly to pay these food costs. Lawton states:

> A perhaps over-simplified summary of past experience leads us to state that the only way meals can be provided without subsidy is to make mandatory the taking of all or a majority of meals in the common dining room. This, of course, drives the cost of the housing package up to a point where another segment of the elderly population is priced out of the possibility of living there. [82]

He worries that "for the most part only luxury retirement centers can provide all three meals, since there is no satisfactory way that this can be done utilizing a single eight hour work shift."[83]

There is an urgent need to see that the cost of these meals is not entirely borne by the tenant and the development, for otherwise congregate housing cannot be made available to low-income elderly. And if it is not, the situation of pushing elderly into nursing homes who could be housed in congregate developments will continue, and the higher per person cost to the state will continue. As the state of Maryland Office on Aging has pointed out in budgeting for state support of the food package in sheltered housing, a rationale for such funding is "the offset gained in leveling off and minimizing payments in Medicaid for nursing home care."[84]

Some, such as Thompson, [85] argue that the federal government must make a commitment to fund some of these food costs. Specifically, some, such as Kallia Bokser, coordinator of services of the New York City Housing Authority, feel HUD must move from its role as a "somewhat remote negotiator and adviser to that of an active participant."[86] These spokesmen for congregate housing want more assurance rather than the present short-term agreements with AOA or other sources, that funding of any meal service will continue. [87]

Developments that are congregate have resorted to a number of ways to try to lower food costs. Some have a self-service buffet-type breakfast, thereby attempting to avoid a double kitchen shift. Residents may be used to set this up, just as in some developments they are used to set the table, prepare food, and such, thus lowering costs of staff. The development may have cafeteria style for all meals to cut staff costs. The problem with this, as with a buffet breakfast, is that it is hard for the more handicapped elderly to use this service, as we found in our observed Minnesota congregate housing (Berkshire Home in Osseo). Someone must specially look after disable residents, or a waitress service must be used for all. A compromise for the main meals is that dessert and possibly appetizer be served cafeteria style, with the well elderly helping the disabled, and then the main course be served by staff.

As for cutting cost by making meals compulsory, many congregate developments do this, though apartment developments serving a noon meal only usually do not. Some experts feel the elderly should be given a choice as to whether they take meals; however, this unpredictability of number of meals to serve, plus accounting costs, increases the total meal cost. And poorer residents, who may need the meals, will opt not to take them due to cost.

Choice of a main course, while again lessening the institutional atmosphere, can only be done cheaply if the second choice is a standard alternative that is easy to prepare and cheap. However, one must usually serve special meals to those with special dietary needs. In general the food should meet the standard dietary allowance often worked out by a staff or community agency dietician. Since food is a major complaint in any congregate development, as found in our study, attempts at creativity are worth the effort.

One may also get more satisfied tenants if some of their peers serve on a food committee of the tenant association and help to plan meals within the limits of the meal budget. If they are a special ethnic group, they may help the management decide on ethnic preferences. The tenants will then better realize the alternatives in keeping food costs low.

One cost cutter is to use a catering service and then use a minimal number of staff. Another is not to serve meals on Sunday, staff's day off, or to only serve hot noon meals and have cold evening meals, thus letting some kitchen staff out of work early.

In taking any of these cost-saving steps, the management should watch to see that they do not in a major way contribute an institutional look or detract from the image of dining being a warm, pleasant experience. Dining room users in our study complained about overly regimented dining room hours, something that can easily be corrected. They also complained of overcrowding in the dining room and insufficient dining room staff, both matters that can be worked out. They also complained of lack of provision for special diets, indicating a greater need for kitchen staff sensitive to the needs of the elderly. Dining room staff also must be made sensitive to such elderly needs as help in eating and problems arising from some residents' confusion and senility. Since the help are often from a minority group, while the residents are white, training on these needs is all the more important to avoid hostilities, which can again make dining an unpleasant experience rather than the high point of the day that it should be.

Housekeeping and Personal Care Services

Housekeeping and homemaker services are required by the somewhat impaired and frail elderly in developments. These elderly no longer have the energy to do housework or they are marginally competent, too confused, in doing it. In our user study, almost a third said they had difficulty doing everyday housework, making beds, washing, and cleaning the room. While 58, or most of these, were in congregate housing and of course received such help, 32 having difficulty were in apartments. Of these 32 (17 percent of the surveyed apartment dwellers) having difficulty, only three used a homemaker service.

Problems with housekeeping were in fact a reason some had come to the development. Indeed, 16 percent said they had come to the development because of need for help in homemaking, cooking, and shopping, and another 27 percent because they were unable to keep up the maintenance of their own home.

In a large survey of residents in elderly public housing without services, Lawton[88] found there was a very high level of support for the availability of assistance with housekeeping and personal care. He reported that "while the majority of tenants did not feel such a need for themselves at that time, they clearly would feel more secure knowing that it was available should they need it, and they also were wholly in favor of its being available to others who did require help."[89]

Some development managers say they only select tenants who can do their own housekeeping. However, the need for help can arise for these tenants after they have been in the housing several years.

The degree of need may vary with the health conditions of the residents. First, many in apartments and even in congregate housing may be well enough to do their housework and to make beds. The need may be just for help in heavy work, such as vacuuming, waxing floors, cleaning windows. Second, some in both apartments and congregate housing, if they need more complete housekeeping help, may only need it on a weekly basis while others are so incompetent or in such poor health that they need it on a daily basis. It may be that the service is only temporarily needed, when the person is ill and/or returns from the hospital. For example, in a Niagara Falls, New York, elderly public housing development,[90] the housekeeping unit helps those who have just returned from the hospital with changing the linen, cooking the meals, and taking care of personal needs, according to a tenant leader there.

Because different tenants, both in apartments and congregate housing, have different needs, there is a controversy, not only over how often the service should be supplied—daily, weekly, or on call— but over how to supply it and how it should be paid for.

Some experts suggest that tenants have an option on whether they want the service daily or weekly, and they be charged accordingly. If a fee is charged, it is argued, only those who need the service will sign up for it, while if it is free, all will, and this unneces-

sarily increases the cost to the development. This method of limit-
ing use may also answer Thompson's worry[91] that in providing the
service one can easily create an air of dependency, make the development more of a nursing home, and of course increase cost. She feels
in providing the service one has to determine if the person really
needs it. However, if one uses a fee as a means of determining this,
the problem if that poorer tenants in need will possibly not request
it. A number of developments do charge fees instead of including
the cost in the monthly rent for congregate housing; for example, in
the congregate wing of the Burwell, Nebraska, elderly housing in 1975,
those unable to do their own housework could contract for a housekeeping service they paid for; a homemaker also came in to bathe one
tenant. Some developments use elderly tenants, either in a volunteer
or paid capacity, to help the few tenants in need of housekeeping assistance.

   Community homemaker services are used in a number of developments. In most subsidized apartment developments, if their tenants
have any assistance in housekeeping, they have it through this source.
Almost 40 percent of our surveyed apartment managers said homemaker service was available to their development; another 4 percent
said it was an on-site service provided by the development (see Table
6.4). Few surveyed apartment dwellers in 19 developments in the
user survey said they used a homemaker service; only three of 116
apartment dwellers said they did.

   Whether the service is weekly or daily housekeeping or homemaker assistance, the personnel involved are on the front line in
helping tenants in crises and in alerting the management to such; they
also are a regular social contact source for the residents.

Personal Care Services

   Personal care services—grooming, dressing, bathing, and personal hygiene services; hair, skin, and foot care; clothes care; and
minor exercising—are often performed by the same staff that handles
the housekeeping tasks. Sometimes some of these personal care responsibilities, such as bathing and foot care, are performed by
nurse's aides. These services are again for the less competent elderly who may have handicaps such as arthritis that make it hard for
them to dress themselves, or loss of memory and confusion that
mean they have similar needs. They may be so depressed that they
neglect their personal hygiene and their apartment. The elderly in
need may have just returned from the hospital or be temporarily ill,
and for a short time have to be helped. Many others, especially
in congregate housing, have a permanent need.

   If these personal needs for daily living can be taken care of,
these elderly can be kept out of a nursing home. A person may have

TABLE 6.4

Availability of Services, by Rural–Urban Areas

Service	Metropolitan		Other Urban		Rural		Total	
	Number	Percent	Number	Percent	Number	Percent	Number	Percent
Home nursing assistance								
Available	89	85.5	24	88.9	87	53.3	200	68.0
Not available	9	8.7	2	7.4	63	38.7	74	25.2
No answer	6	5.8	1	3.7	13	8.0	20	6.8
Homemaker service								
Available	62	59.6	10	37.0	32	19.6	104	35.4
Not available	31	29.8	14	51.9	108	66.3	153	52.0
No answer	11	10.6	3	11.1	23	14.1	37	12.6
Prepared meal delivery service								
Available	61	58.7	17	63.0	22	13.5	100	34.0
Not available	31	29.8	9	33.3	129	79.1	169	57.5
No answer	12	11.5	1	3.7	12	7.4	25	8.5

Source: Canadian manager survey.

147

only one of the abovementioned needs and it may be minor, so that it
can be taken care of once a week or less frequently. Moreover, it is
assumed only a proportion of all the residents in the congregate development will need the personal care services. This will depend on
selection of tenants and how long they have been in the development.
If the number needing help is small, the development may feel they
can handle these residents' needs even when the needs become extensive, rather than sending these persons on to a nursing home. If the
number is small, the development might have its housekeeper staff
handle the personal care need or rely on community homemaker services in the case of an apartment development; the community visiting
nurse may bathe residents, as was true at several of our studied developments; or the development may, again, use residents as voluntee
or paid personal care staff to help the few residents in need; however,
some residents may not want to take on the job of helping incompetent
or sick residents as it reminds them of their own possible fate. In
our observed Minneapolis area development (Berkshire Home in Osseo) a resident did do ironing to earn pin money.

Personal Care Facilities

A laundry is an important facility in any development as it means
easy access to a necessary clothes care source. Even in many congregate developments, tenants or their relatives must wash their own
sheets and towels, although personal aides may see that this is done
by the development for certain impaired residents. However, in congregate developments where many are impaired or are middle class,
the development may do this.

The laundry also serves another function. It is a meeting place
where social contacts, especially in apartment developments, are established. Almost all developments included in our manager survey
had laundries. The few that did not were congregate developments
that took care of this service for residents, either having a staff member run a development laundry or sending laundry out to a commercial
firm. In a few cases there was a laundry within five blocks. In the
user survey, all users had a laundry available to them and 83 percent
of these surveyed residents used it. Many of those who did not were
in congregate developments. The major complaint from users was
that the machine frequently broke down, a complaint mentioned in all
developments. Other complaints were "no dryer," "coin operated,"
"inconvenient schedule for use," "don't know how to use it," and "no
outside clothesline."

Beauty shops and barber shops are other personal care facilities
that can be especially useful in inaccessible outer area developments
or in developments where many of the residents have health limita-

tions. Care of one's hair gives one a feeling of pride and respect, while neglect of hair not only has a negative psychological impact on the person, but, when many residents do not keep up their hair, presents a depressing environment, with tenants looking more like they are in a nursing home. Often these beauty and barber facilities are manned by an outside operator on a certain day or days.

Many congregate developments, especially those serving a middle-class clientele, have a beauty shop and barber shop on the site. A third of the congregate and mixed developments in our manager study had a beauty shop on site and about an equal proportion had a barber shop on site. Only 2 percent of the apartment developments had a beauty shop on site and few had a barber shop. A very large proportion of the developments that did not have a beauty shop or barber shop on site had one available within five blocks. However, for all developments, almost a third did not have a beauty shop accessible (with 5 blocks) and an equally large share did not have a barber shop accessible; many of these were apartment developments.

There is always a question whether one should provide the space for such facilities and then encourage professionals to staff them, for use is often low (partly due to the expense), and, with barber service, the number of male residents available to use it is low. In our user survey, two-thirds of these elderly said hairdressing (barber/beauty shop) was available in the development, with it more likely to be available in the congregate development; but 40 percent of those who said it was available did not use the service. The reasons they did not use it were "do own hair," "go to another shop," and "too expensive." These problems with supplying the service may be the reason why in the manager survey very few of the managers who did not have an on-site beauty shop felt the need for one, with a very small proportion of apartment managers feeling the need and only a third of the managers of congregate housing feeling the need.

STAFFING

If housing for the elderly is going to be a supportive environment, it needs to be staffed. Many elderly see the staff providing a source of assistance in times of emergency or temporary needs. This is especially true if the elderly have no relatives in the area; our study showed that half of the 44 percent of the elderly sample who said they would turn to the development staff, versus families, in times of emergency, had no relatives in the area. Existence of staff provides a feeling of security. In developments where staff is lacking, especially on weekends and in evenings, the elderly feel uneasy because they fear lack of help for emergency illnesses or lack of vigilance against intruders. As elderly in our survey pointed out, they might fall in their apartment and no one might discover it for several days.

The most likely staff is composed of the manager and the maintenance man. However, one hopes that if the services mentioned above are to be provided by the development itself, at least part-time staff would be hired to cover these tasks. If the services are to be provided by the community instead, staff of other agencies visit the development on a regular basis. If the development is of the congregate type or a mix of congregate and apartments, then usually more staff will be required as the impaired elderly in congregate units have more need for supportive services.

Questions about staffing include the size of the staff needed for different-size developments, the type of staff needed, and the duties of this staff. While size of staff will vary with size and type of development, a fundamental concern is that there be some staff present to give support to these elderly users. In our Canadian survey of developments we found about a fifth of the apartment developments had no on-site staff and most of the others had two or fewer staff persons; even many of the very large developments had only one person or no staff. With this situation, it is not surprising that, when asked about satisfaction with staff, many in our sample of apartment users said they were bothered by shortage of staff.

Some housing authorities have one management staff for several projects. Some have a central maintenance staff instead of on-site staff. Some nonprofit sponsors of small developments simply have a board that, through monthly meetings and volunteer work, such as rent collecting and account keeping, manages the small project.

Most congregate and mixed developments in contrast had three or more staff members. In the apartment developments the most likely staff member was not the manager but the maintenance man. Almost all apartment developments had a maintenance man and only about 13 percent had a manager (this is the proportion for the developments for which responses to this question were given, but since there were 49 nonresponses to the question, which might in reality be no responses, the proportion having no manager may be higher). In general terms the fact is that for the apartment developments, well over three-fourths had either no staff or only a maintenance man.

In some housing authorities, such as metropolitan Toronto, the maintenance men at the time of the study were told by the authority that their role was not a social service role and they were not to fulfill this function for their tenants or even indulge in much contact with the tenants. In the National Center for Housing Management manual[93] for managers of elderly, this line of thinking is also put forth; maintenance men are considered not to be doing a good job if they spend time filling tenants' requests and communicating with tenants, as illustrated in one of the manual's case studies. Attitudes vary however; in metropolitan Toronto in 1974 the authority changed its attitudes toward the role of maintenance men, realizing they were the only regular staff in the elderly apartment developments and thus the only ones who had direct contact with the elderly. In 1974 metropolitan Toronto was considering expanding the role of the caretaker to help provide on-site community services.[94] In 1974 the authority had one caretaker for every building, with the building often having 300-350 units; this caretaker is only on duty during the day. A few buildings also had a night security guard. Even if the maintenance man takes on resident contact services, the question is whether he has the time and is qualified to do it. For example, for the very large Ontario Housing Corporation, where social service work is part of their job, the complaint has been that caretakers are overworked and not able to help residents as much as they are expected to in this authority. This is not surprising since the caretaker covers 300-500 units; he is backed up by five building service or community care workers as auxiliary support or supervisory staff, usually out of the main office, for every 700 units.

Our feeling is that the maintenance staff, because of the nonexistence or shortage of alternative staff, should take on tenant contacts and be trained to convey elderly needs they observe or to communicate emergency needs to the appropriate social service personnel in the downtown housing authority office or, in case of medical needs, to the appropriate emergency medical resource. As Thompson[95] says, the maintenance man can be as important as the manager to the elderly residents, providing informal friendships, quick and expert service, and a friendly greeting. But these maintenance men should not, on the other hand, be used as a substitute manager.

Thompson assumes there will be a manager in apartment developments. However, in the United States, as in Canada, on-site staff is sometimes not found, though these cases are decreasing. In some places in both the United States and Canada, the British warden system[96] is used either to supplement the day staff with evening live-in staff or as the only staff. For example, the San Francisco Housing Authority had live-in college students for several years: they got their apartment free. In Britain, where the local authority's elderly housing is often in clusters of 30 dwellings, the live-in wardens cover responsibilities of a very limited kind; the main job is general oversight of the complex of mainly well elderly and availability for the occasional emergency, sometimes in terms of responding to the alarm system that exists in each unit. Usually a couple is used, with the husband in outside employment and the wife taking on the warden responsibilities. In Britain the couple receive a free flat and possibly part-time pay, according to John Macey, former head of Greater London Council housing.[97] While there have been cases where college students or other couples have not been as reliable as one would like, this is one partial solution to night and weekend staff coverage. There is no question that the statistics show in both Canada and the United States that this coverage is lacking and is a concern to the elderly user and to many experts. In other chapters we have indicated that with residents' long stay in these apartments, their health conditions are worsening. In the United States experts say we have a crisis in elderly public housing because many elderly need supportive services, including occasional medical assistance. In Canada, for 15 of our surveyed apartment complexes with few or no staff persons, the health status of over half of the residents was "some incapacity." This means assistance may be needed and emergencies may arise. Where is the staff to handle them?

Besides assuming there will be a manager in all developments, Lawton[98] suggests, for what he calls "bare minimum service level" in elderly housing complexes, a weekly visit from a nurse. In our Canadian study a few apartment developments had office staff (15 did) and a very few had housekeeping, kitchen, religious, nursing, auxiliary medical, or occupational therapy staff (see Tables 6.5 and 6.6). Missing in both Canadian housing and in U.S. recommendations are a social work staff or recreational staff for apartment developments. We do know that in some middle-class elderly apartment developments these are found. In many cases it is assumed the manager or assistant manager, if there is one, will take on these duties. In most U.S. public housing complexes the central housing authority's office staff includes community service personnel who fill this function for all its developments or a set number. HUD assumes that their job as well as the manager's, in the area of social services, is mainly to contact the community service agencies[99] and get them to relate to the elderly population. Some such agencies do in some areas provide staff specifically to the housing development, as already mentioned.

Congregate developments usually have many more staff persons as they are providing such services as housekeeping, meals, and minimal nursing care. In our study only one congregate or mixed development reporting on staff has less than three staff persons, with most having six or more and almost two-thirds of them having 15 or more. Developments serving a residential clientele where half or more of the residents had an incapacity usually had a high number of personnel.

Size of the facility of course had an effect on the size of the staff. Moreover, some of the nonprofit developments run by nuns had a larger staff.

Almost all these developments had a manager, at least one maintenance man, and a kitchen and a housekeeping staff. Half had

TABLE 6.5

Availability of Development Personnel, Total

Personnel	1 or More All Part Time	1, Full Time	2, at Least 1 Full Time	3-4, at Least 1 Full Time	5 and Over, at Least 1 Full Time	None	No Answer	Total
Administrative								
Number	10	48	23	8	3	151	51	294
Percent	3.4	16.3	7.8	2.8	1.0	51.4	17.3	100
Maintenance/security								
Number	81	60	34	28	8	34	49	294
Percent	27.6	20.4	11.6	9.4	2.7	11.6	16.7	100
Office								
Number	13	29	6	2	1	193	50	294
Percent	4.4	9.9	2.0	0.7	0.4	65.6	17.0	100
Religious								
Number	2	10	0	4	0	227	51	294
Percent	0.7	3.4	0.0	1.4	0.0	77.2	17.3	100
Kitchen								
Number	0	5	7	34	28	168	52	294
Percent	0.0	1.7	2.4	11.6	9.5	57.1	17.7	100
Housekeeping								
Number	1	8	6	28	29	171	51	294
Percent	0.3	2.7	2.0	9.6	9.9	58.2	17.3	100
Doctor								
Number	1	0	0	0	0	237	56	294
Percent	0.3	0.0	0.0	0.0	0.0	80.7	19.0	100
Nurses								
Number	6	21	6	10	11	189	51	294
Percent	2.0	7.1	2.0	3.5	3.7	64.4	17.3	100
Auxiliary medical								
Number	6	5	0	8	21	202	52	294
Percent	2.0	1.7	0.0	2.7	7.2	68.7	17.7	100
Occupational therapists								
Number	7	1	0	0	0	235	51	294
Percent	2.4	0.3	0.0	0.0	0.0	80.0	17.3	100

Source: Canadian manager survey.

TABLE 6.6

Availability of Development Personnel, by Self-Contained Apartments

Personnel	1 or More, All Part Time	1, Full Time	2, at Least 1 Full Time	3-4, at Least 1 Full Time	5 and Over, at Least 1 Full Time	None	No Answer	Total
Administrative								
Number	9	11	2	0	0	149	49	220
Percent	4.1	5.0	0.9	0.0	0.0	67.7	22.3	100
Maintenance/security								
Number	78	37	16	10	2	30	47	220
Percent	35.5	16.8	7.3	4.5	0.9	13.6	21.4	100
Religious								
Number	1	1	0	2	0	167	49	220
Percent	0.5	0.5	0.0	0.9	0.0	75.9	22.3	100
Kitchen								
Number	0	1	0	3	0	167	49	220
Percent	0.0	0.5	0.0	1.4	0.0	75.8	22.3	100
Housekeeping								
Number	0	1	0	3	1	166	49	220
Percent	0.0	0.5	0.0	1.4	0.5	75.3	22.3	100
Doctors								
Number	0	0	0	0	0	169	51	220
Percent	0.0	0.0	0.0	0.0	0.0	76.8	23.2	100
Nurses								
Number	2	0	0	0	0	169	49	220
Percent	0.9	0.0	0.0	0.0	0.0	76.8	22.3	100
Auxiliary medical								
Number	2	0	0	0	0	169	49	220
Percent	0.9	0.0	0.0	0.0	0.0	76.8	22.3	100
Occupational therapists								
Number	2	0	0	0	0	169	49	220
Percent	0.9	0.0	0.0	0.0	0.0	76.8	22.3	100
Office								
Number	9	6	0	0	0	157	48	220
Percent	4.1	2.7	0.0	0.0	0.0	71.4	21.8	100

Source: Canadian manager survey.

office staff. Over two-thirds had at least one nurse, with most having two; some of these (18 of the 52 having a nurse) had a nursing wing. Half had auxiliary medical staff as well. However, only one congregate development had a doctor on staff. Only a few had an occupational therapist or religious staff.

Thompson[100] in 1975 suggested that for every 100 congregate units, one should have a full-time trained resident manager, a clerical person, an engineer-maintenance superintendent and one helper, two part-time housekeepers-matrons, and one part-time landscaper-janitorial assistant.

HUD 1972 guidelines for congregate housing[101] (now being revised) were less generous, recommending only a part-time manager, a clerical person, an engineer and helper, and only one matron-housekeeper or personal aide. We feel this is far too small a staff to serve an impaired elderly population that otherwise might go into a nursing home where the ratio of staff to patients is astronomically greater. HUD regulations did recommend these positions be full time if the complex had 100-200 units; they then recommend two housekeepers. For developments of 300 units and over they did recommend adding a human services coordinator and increasing the number of housekeepers. They in fact suggest larger projects have a small staff of social service personnel as part of the total management team. They make no mention of a nurse. These guidelines suggest the development with minimum staff rely on volunteers such as housewives and college students or the elderly themselves for seasonally required or one-time functions. While we found nonprofit developments where the sponsoring group helped with landscaping, gardening, and carpentry work, or provided special parties for residents, this assistance was often sporadic and could not be relied on. Only 7 percent of our surveyed developments had volunteers put in more than ten hours a week, and no public housing did. Managers told us they got little help from service clubs or from church groups.

Health personnel are not emphasized in the HUD 1972 guidelines or by Thompson,[102] but Lawton[103] feels "moderate level" housing for marginally competent tenants should have 24-hour telephone access to a nurse employed by the housing project and daily visits by a doctor. It should also have an activity program directed by a designated professional and paid for either by the sponsor or a community organization. It should also have a part-time on-site social worker or other trained personnel to provide personal and social counseling. Lawton does not mention housekeeping staff.

For his "maximum services" housing for relatively dependent elderly, a type of development that resembles many congregate complexes, Lawton[104] advises daily nurse's and doctor's hours, thus assuming staff, a full-time counselor for social and personal counseling, a professional directing the activities program, as well as personal grooming-housekeeping-laundry assistance and meal service personnel. Lawton's inclusion[105] of nursing staff and activities program and social-personal counseling staff comes closer to what we feel is needed or what is found in some of our surveyed Canadian congregate developments, which did provide nursing staff, though they skimped on social work and recreational staff. The need for some nursing staff to fill minor medical needs, but not to take on the job of the nursing home nurse, seems useful and something desired by the elderly themselves. Activities and social work staff can help the elderly to adjust to this new home, to participate in activities, and to get help for their legal, financial, and health problems. We know a number of nonprofit congregate developments that do have such staff. For example, the Berkshire Home outside Minneapolis has nurses as managers and some social activities staff. Some centers have recreational staff because they are headquarters for the neighborhood's elderly activities. For example, Park View Plaza in Burwell, Nebraska,[106] which has congregate units and apartments, has Title III funding for an areawide recreation and craft program headquartered in their development. The Our Lady congregate development in Oakland, California, also houses a senior center for the area, and staff is provided for this.

The type of staff and number cannot relate only to what the community is supplying but to the conditions of the elderly. In some congregate housing most residents are well while in other developments many are senile, have problems walking, need medication, or have other health problems.

There is some justification for suggesting either "add-on" programs and staff, as resident needs increase, as Carp says,[107] or a flexible staff arrangement as the HUD guidelines suggest. They say:

> Since congregate housing will, in many ways and in varying degrees, be "flexible housing," to take care of the needs of a diverse clientele with personal needs and support differing in degree or length of time, the staffing for the administrative and maintenance functions must also be flexible. Determining staff standards, both number and character, is difficult. Many non-profit organizations and sponsors manage elements of the programs themselves, using their own resources in addition to or apart from the formal or paid staff. Direction is necessary, however, to provide a yardstick against which to measure adequacy and overall costs. The goal is the retention of the residential character of the building while providing supportive services as needed, related to institutional concepts.

Institutional costs are higher and emphasis should be on
the minimum to assure resident care as required.[108]

Role of the Manager

The job of the manager, whether in apartment or congregate
developments, must be a flexible one. In most developments it is
assumed he will be an administrator who supervises the staff and
takes overall responsibility for all the many aspects of management,
including supervision of maintenance work and handling of a variety
of fiscal matters including rent collection, payment of bills, often
with the help of an accountant or office worker. The manager must
get involved in hiring personnel, paying attention to security, and
even handling legal aspects. One of his biggest jobs may be record
keeping and report writing, as Lawton[109] found in his survey of U.S.
public housing managers.

In our survey most managers (78 percent of all), but more nonprofit managers, said one of their main jobs was keeping accounts
and managing the finances for the development; about the same proportion said collecting the rent was their main responsibility. Almost two-thirds said maintenance was also presently their job or
should be "very much" their responsibility; over three-fourths of
the public housing managers said this. These managers were much
less likely to say that running social service programs or obtaining
community services was presently their job (or to feel it should be
"very much" their responsibility). Public housing managers were
especially reluctant to say these jobs were their responsibility, with
only 35 percent of public housing managers, versus 46 percent of
nonprofit managers, saying obtaining community services was presently their job or feeling it should be "very much" their responsibility;
only 16 percent of public housing managers, versus 31 percent of
nonprofit managers, said running social service programs was presently their job or felt it "very much" should be their responsibility
(see Table 6.7).

These managers were somewhat more likely to include helping
residents with needs on an individual basis as presently their job or
say it should be "very much" their responsibility; 55 percent of those
in each group responded yes, that it was their job. Yet this means
many did not have as their job, or feel it should be their job, what
we consider a basic obligation, helping the residents. This contrasts
with the responses of Lawton's sample of U.S. public housing managers
who said one of their two main jobs was "direct contact with the tenants."

In general we also must conclude, regarding these Canadian managers, that they neither had as their job nor felt they should have as part of their job these social service and tenant contact functions.

For Lawton's sample, besides the other major job of record keeping, jobs of lesser importance and taking less time were supervision of other staff, dealing with the sponsors, and, even less, talking to relatives of tenants.

There has been a great interest in expanding the manager's duties to include responsibilities related to helping to meet client nonhousing needs. The effort is to move the manager away from the model of being strictly a building manager who also handles fiscal matters.

Lawton[110] suggests the manager take on an information and referral role and be a counselor to the elderly. Thompson[111] sees coordination of a variety of services as the major role besides fiscal management. For congregate housing, she elaborates this role as including development of a tenant selection or placement plan, management of an essential services program of food, housekeeping, and personal services, activation of a social program, and work on tenant relations. She also includes knowledge and use of community resources development and a specific medical resource program.

The HUD 1972 guidelines for congregate housing[112] stress that besides management of rent collection and business office, other management responsibilities are making contact with the community resources and fostering community relations, possibly preoccupancy interviews for residents, though this may be done by a special staff, and work with a resident council.

In its manual for managers of elderly housing, the National Center for Housing Management[113] devotes chapters to the manager's role. The role includes responsibility in the areas of security, money, legal rights, personnel, maintenance, and promoting the apartment and social services, according to the manual. It devotes very little space to the manager's role in providing social services, feeling these services should mainly come from the community.

It is our opinion that the manager should take a major part in seeing that supportive services are provided, either by the development or the community, and a major role in contact with the tenants so that he knows their needs and can take on an advocacy referral role with the residents as well as an advocacy role in obtaining community services. He cannot limit his tasks to that of a simple building superintendent, as found in middle-class city apartments, ignoring the special needs of the elderly tenant group.

The manager of congregate housing will have more roles to play than the apartment manager. Thompson sees these managers of congregate housing needing training and educational background for their roles. She says:

TABLE 6.7

Degree to Which Duties of Development Staff Respondents Include Obtaining Community Services, by Rural-Urban Areas

	Metropolitan		Other Urban		Rural		Total	
	Number	Percent	Number	Percent	Number	Percent	Number	Percent
Manager answering								
Presently my job	15	14.4	5	18.5	29	17.8	49	16.7
Should be my job	6	5.8	2	7.4	28	17.2	36	12.2
Should not be my job	10	9.6	6	22.2	29	17.8	45	15.3
Sponsor answering								
Presently my job	2	1.9	0	0.0	10	6.2	12	4.1
Should be my job	3	2.9	0	0.0	7	4.3	10	3.4
Should not be my job	13	12.6	1	3.8	0	0.0	14	4.8
Other staff answering								
Presently my job	15	14.4	3	11.1	3	1.8	21	7.1
Should be my job	0	0.0	0	0.0	1	0.6	1	0.3
Should not be my job	2	1.9	0	0.0	2	1.2	4	1.4
No answer	38	36.5	10	37.0	54	33.1	102	34.7

Source: Canadian manager survey.

From this brief sketch of the management role and function,
it is clear that congregate housing is much more than shelter . . . the everyday roles of congregate housing management will require counseling, social intervention, and de-
cision-making based on a better than average knowledge of
gerontology, social medicine and the legal system. Fiscal management and coordination of the variety of services
also will require expertise beyond that now practiced in
the management housing for the hale and hearty elderly
capable of living completely independent lives.[114]

Whether managers are trained and oriented to all these roles
is questionable. Many seem to be struggling with problems in a number of these areas. For example, tenant relations was given by a
large group of managers in our study as their biggest problem; it was
the third most mentioned problem. Tenant relations, including the
problem of demanding relatives and impolite tenants, was given as a
very major reason for dissatisfaction, again indicating a problem,
in Lawton's survey of managers of such housing. In our manager
study finances, including budgeting, was by far the most major problem, with administrative problems second, and the tenant health
problems and staffing problems also mentioned. These all indicate
the need for more training and education in the role. Other major
dissatisfactions Lawton's[115] surveyed managers had, that is, poor
pay and too much pressure and too much work, indicate other needs.
Reasons for satisfaction given by managers in Lawton's study illus-
trate why personnel might want to get the training to better perform
the social work and counseling part of this job; these reasons for
satisfaction were "helping other people" and "gratitude expressed by
tenants."
        This need for training is beginning to be met. The National
Center for Housing Management has run courses on housing the elderly, as have some academic institutions. NAHRO has pushed for such
training and HUD has backed up their interest with funding to various
groups.
        The kinds of training required center around making the mana-
ger especially aware of the needs of the elderly group and of the
ways he can make their life more comfortable. As Thompson says,
training for the manager of congregate housing should include "a
scientific understanding of the aging process as a basis of program-
ming; experience in handling health emergencies, providing first aid
and quickly securing pre-arranged professional assistance around the
clock."[116] Maybe is managers have training in these aspects, tenants will not give as their reason for dissatisfaction with the development, as in our user survey they did, "need better prepared staff to
handle residents' problems and need changes in management policies."

At present most managers have not had such training. In fact, in Lawton's[117] survey of public housing and Section 202 managers he found only half had attended a training course or conference on problems of managing housing for the elderly; even more distressing, as it shows their lack of interest, very few of these managers belonged to any organization in the field. Lawton found less than 1 percent of these public housing managers had worked with the elderly before taking this job.

In our survey of Canadian managers we found a somewhat better situation. Over half the managers had worked with the elderly for five or more years; another fourth had worked with them two to four years and only 15 percent had worked with them less than two years. Public housing managers were less likely than nonprofit housing managers to have worked with the elderly for five or more years. Managers of metropolitan area developments were much more likely to have worked with the elderly five or more years than was true for managers of rural or other urban area housing.

As for education, well over half our surveyed Canadian managers had some college education and over a fourth had three or more years of college. In Lawton's survey of U.S. managers they also typically had some college education, and one-fourth of the public housing managers and 40 percent of the Section 202 managers were college graduates.

Other Staff

Other staff besides the manager and maintenance men may be wardens or auxiliary apartment staff, such as an assistant manager, who act as receptionists, office staff, and contact personnel. Their main job may be to complement the manager in terms of 24-hour coverage. The emergency call system in the elderly person's apartment or room may be connected to an apartment manned by this staff who get the apartment free as part of their job. Such attendance or surveillance of this 24-hour alarm system provides the tenants with a feeling of trust and security. If there is not staff to man such a 24-hour system, there should be arrangements to have the system connect up with a hospital or central office or doctor's office or even the local fire department, as in one case we studied.

The tenants themselves may be recruited to aid in these jobs either as paid staff or volunteers; sometimes they can see the needs of other tenants quicker than development staff. In a number of developments their type of surveillance is part of a buddy system, with the person covering either a whole floor or being one or several persons on that floor. Those recruited are usually the more alert and well elderly. For example, in the Halifax housing we studied (Northwood Towers) one tenant acted as a welcoming committee, ombudsman, and contact for all the elderly residents. In other developments there was a floor manager or buddy system, though some were not very active.

Residents may take on other development tasks, whether as paid or unpaid staff. In fact, such hiring of staff has been recommended. In our Canadian study, nonprofit developments, but not public housing developments, made considerable use of residents. In well over half of the nonprofit developments residents took on such chores as cleaning halls, gardening, or helping out in the kitchen; in most developments less than half of the residents took on these tasks.

In the United States, in some public housing projects the elderly residents have been hired as assistant maintenance men, as receptionists, or as kitchen help. For example, in the Alma, Georgia, Housing Authority's[118] congregate housing the tenants work in the kitchen (after obtaining a health certificate), helping prepare fresh vegetables for meals or for the freezer, including shelling peas, snapping beans, and such. The authority also uses youth workers hired under a federal employment program for gardening work. In one San Francisco public housing project for the elderly a resident cooks hot meals for the elderly once a week. In fact, in one study, in two-thirds of the public housing projects having the Title VII nutrition-meals program, tenants helped prepare the meals. In a Satellite Homes nonprofit development in Oakland, California, an elderly person acts as an assistant manager and 24-hour surveillance person, and in a Burwell, Nebraska, congregate development an elderly tenant is also available to answer the alarm system if a resident needs help. In fact such staffing is rather common. In addition, Lawton[119] found that, in the Section 202 housing surveyed, many managers were retirees especially recruited for the job; over half were 55 and over.

Local housing authorities have the ability to hire residents for a number of jobs in the project under Title X of the Public Works and Economic Development Act of 1965, according to Silverman of HUD.[120] As of 1975 a few authorities had done so. The new Title XX social security program suggests use of personnel for chore services to the elderly and that these personnel can be the elderly themselves.

The HUD handbook on community services functions in the area offices[121] says one objective should be to increase the training and employment of residents in project operations.

Tenants themselves are calling for tenant-run services in public housing. One Canadian tenant leader suggested "the gradual integration of the tenant into the services, that is, kitchen and dining room service, housekeeping units, and minor maintenance duties."[122]

Social Workers

Social workers are another suggested staff. The 1972 HUD guidelines for congregate housing[123] suggest such staff and others have felt they should be included in congregate housing staff. However, few subsidized developments have such staff; a number of authorities do have a central community services staff, as do HUD area offices.

These social workers can be useful in establishing links with community agencies, using advocacy techniques to get residents to make use of community or development services, providing technical assistance to the resident council and, of course, doing individual counseling. (Their duties were described in more detail under the services section.)

While many persons will say the manager can take on these social work jobs, especially the community referral work, many managers, first, have limited time and, second, do not see it as an important part of their job.

A third of our surveyed managers, when asked, said "obtaining community services" should not be part of their job (only 43 percent had it as their job). Almost a fifth of the surveyed managers said "helping residents on a personal basis" should not be part of their job; however, slightly over half said it was part of their job. On the other hand only 5 percent of these managers said there was social work counseling service in the development, whether done by them or others, so we can assume that few help residents on a counseling level.

Housekeepers

In congregate housing another staff group would be housekeepers or matrons. The 1975 HUD congregate guidelines recommended one housekeeping or personal aide for a development with 100-200 residents and three to five such aides for a 300-and-over-unit development. As mentioned above, almost all the congregate developments in the manager study had housekeeping staff and three-fourths had three or more persons in such staff. Twenty of these managers considered housekeeping staff a major problem. Only 2 percent of the surveyed apartments had such staff.

Thompson states some of the diverse opinions on supplying housekeeping staff for congregate developments:

> Here again there are differences of opinion. Some developments feel there should be a daily cleaning as in a hotel, with particular attention to bathroom sanitation. Others

prefer a weekly heavy and thorough cleaning plan. Still others believe the housekeeping service should be available only on request, based on need and individually paid for by the resident. The decision may depend upon the availability of a community housekeeping service and its cost, as well as the level of tenant competence and their paying ability. In developing the operating budget, however, at least the cost of a once a week housekeeping service should be included. In some places, it may be more economical to have staff maids or matrons on a full or part time basis, who also can perform personal services. In other places, itinerant hiring or use of a community housekeeping service may be more economical and quite adequate.[124]

Staffing requirements, as shown above, relate not only to how incompetent the residents are in this area but to whether the service is offered daily or weekly to the tenant and whether it is compulsory for all tenants or given to selective tenants either free or on a fee basis. This may depend on the congregate housing's budget; middle-class developments often have considerable staff in this area, possibly because such residents expect it. Whatever schedule is used, tenants should be made aware of it so they are prepared.

Housekeeping staffing is complicated because, first, in some congregate developments personal care assistance, such as grooming, bathing, and clothes care for the residents, is combined with housekeeping tasks, using one staff. Second, in some developments maintenance men do heavy housework such as polishing floors and cleaning windows. In some developments they use volunteers, usually residents, to help those who temporarily need help.

Recreation Staff

Recreation or activities staff is also needed in congregate developments and to a lesser degree in apartment developments. Its job is to instigate daily activities these elderly residents can take part in, such as the various programs mentioned previously under services. Sometimes this staff is provided by the central local housing authority office; these community service division workers cover all or a number of developments. Sometimes a community agency such as the city's parks and recreation department or the school district's adult education division will provide the worker. It may be that a neighborhood senior citizen program is run at the development and staff is provided for that, or a day care center is set up at the development, or an ethnic or religious group sponsoring the project holds its social programs at the development.

Lack of staff can mean a facility designed for use is an expensive underutilized piece of space. One such example is in Newark; Senator Williams[125] reports that a new 202-unit project has community rooms unutilized because of lack of staff. HUD's Silverman[126] also reports a community room closed in a project in one state because they could not find the help needed to keep it open. The same thing is true of infirmaries in some places. One of our Canadian developments had such an underutilized facility. Thus when we discuss facilities and services, we must keep in mind that above all we must have staff to utilize these facilities. One is of little use without the other. If nothing else, we must utilize able tenants, student help, even medical interns and student nurses, and youth that can be employed through the public works programs. Staff give a warm feeling, a sense of home, to any development. And they give not only services but a sense of security to elderly residents.

NOTES

1. National Center for Housing Management, Housing for Elderly: The On-Site Housing Manager's Resource Book (Washington, D.C.: National Center for Housing Management, 1974), chap. 9, p. 1.
2. Ibid.
3. Testimony by Robert Notte, director, Newark Redevelopment and Housing Authority, in Adequacy of Federal Response to Housing Needs of Older Americans, Hearings, U.S. Congress, Senate, Special Committee on Aging, 94th Cong., 1st sess., October 1975, pt. 13, p. 911.
4. Frances M. Carp, "Congregate Housing: Concept and Role" (paper presented at National Conference on Congregate Housing for Older People, Washington, D.C., November 11-12, 1975).
5. M. Powell Lawton, Planning and Managing Housing for the Elderly (New York: John Wiley and Sons, 1975).
6. U.S. Department of Housing and Urban Development, HUD Handbook: Community Service Functions in the Area Insuring Office (Washington, D.C.: U.S. Government Printing Office, December 1974).
7. U.S. Department of Housing and Urban Development, Management of Congregate Housing: HUD Guidelines (Washington, D.C.: U.S. Government Printing Office, 1972).
8. "Supportive Services" (paper presented at National Conference on Congregate Housing for Older People, Washington, D.C., November 11-12, 1975).
9. Testimony by Kallia Bokser, coordinator, New York City Public Housing Authority, in Adequacy of Federal Response to Housing Needs of Older Americans, p. 917.

10. Testimony by Louis Danzig, executive secretary, New Jersey Association of Housing and Redevelopment Authorities, in Adequacy of Federal Response to Housing Needs of Older Americans, p. 912.

11. Testimony by Marie McGuire Thompson, Adequacy of Federal Response to Housing Needs of Older Americans, p. 903.

12. Ibid.; Lawton, in Adequacy of Federal Response to Housing Needs of Older Americans, p. 1011.

13. Danzig, in Adequacy of Federal Response to Housing Needs of Older Americans, p. 909.

14. Testimony by Wilma Donahue, in Adequacy of Federal Response to Housing Needs of Older Americans, p. 896.

15. National Center for Housing Management, Housing for Elderly, chap. 9, p. 1.

16. Thomspon, in Adequacy of Federal Response to Housing Needs of Older Americans, p. 903.

17. Arlie Hochschild, "Disengagement Theory: A Critique and Proposal," American Sociological Review 40, no. 5 (October 1975): 553-60; Vern Bengtson, The Social Psychology of Aging (Indianapolis: Bobbs-Merrill, 1973), p. 30.

18. U.S. Department of Housing and Urban Development, HUD Handbook.

19. U.S. Department of Housing and Urban Development, HUD Guidelines.

20. Testimony by Frederic Fay, director, Richmond (Virginia) Redevelopment and Housing Authority, in Adequacy of Federal Response to Housing Needs of Older Americans, pt. 14, p. 1003.

21. Lawton, Planning and Managing Housing for the Elderly, pp. 294-95.

22. Abraham Monk, "The Emergence of Day Care Centers for the Aged: Trends and Planning Issues" (paper presented at National Conference on Social Welfare, Cincinnati, May 1974).

23. Lawton, Planning and Managing Housing for the Elderly, p. 293.

24. "Park View Plaza, Burwell, Nebr.," in Adequacy of Federal Response to Housing Needs of Older Americans, Appendix 6, p. 980.

25. Fay, in Adequacy of Federal Response to Housing Needs of Older Americans, p. 1003.

26. Lawton, Planning and Managing Housing for the Elderly, p. 167.

27. "Congregate Housing Developments in Toledo and Columbus, Ohio," in Adequacy of Federal Response to Housing Needs of Older Americans, Appendix 4, p. 973.

28. Bokser, in Adequacy of Federal Response to Housing Needs of Older Americans, p. 916.

29. U.S. Department of Housing and Urban Development, HUD Handbook; Lawton, Planning and Managing Housing for the Elderly, p. 259.

30. U.S. Department of Housing and Urban Development, HUD Guidelines, p. 18.

31. U.S. Department of Housing and Urban Development, HUD Handbook.

32. Lawton, Planning and Managing Housing for the Elderly, pp. 259-60; Marie McGuire Thompson, "Management of Congregate Housing" (paper presented at National Conference on Congregate Housing for Older People, Washington, D.C., November 11-12, 1975), p. 16.

33. Lawton, Planning and Managing Housing for the Elderly, p. 90.

34. Ibid., p. 110.

35. Testimony by Abner Silverman, counselor to HUD, in Adequacy of Federal Response to Housing Needs of Older Americans, pt. 14, p. 987.

36. Lawton, Planning and Managing Housing for the Elderly, p. 88.

37. Silverman, in Adequacy of Federal Response to Housing Needs of Older Americans, p. 987.

38. Ibid.

39. Testimony by Donald F. Reilly, deputy commissioner, Administration on Aging, in Adequacy of Federal Response to Housing Needs of Older Americans, pt. 14, p. 983.

40. Ibid., p. 985.

41. Donahue, in Adequacy of Federal Response to Housing Needs of Older Americans, pt. 13, p. 896.

42. Ibid.

43. Marie McGuire Thompson, "Congregate Housing for Older Adults: A Working Paper" (presented to U.S. Congress, Senate, Special Committee on Aging, 94th Cong., 1st sess., 1975), p. 26; Lawton, Planning and Managing Housing for the Elderly, p. 302.

44. Testimony by M. Powell Lawton, in Adequacy of Federal Response to Housing Needs of Older Americans, pt. 14, p. 1042.

45. Letter from Patrick J. Feeney, director, Columbus (Ohio) Metropolitan Housing Authority, in Adequacy of Federal Response to Housing Needs of Older Americans, pt. 13, pp. 942-43.

46. U.S. Department of Housing and Urban Development, HUD Guidelines, p. 14.

47. "Interim Guidelines for Sheltered Housing from the Maryland State Office on Aging," in Adequacy of Federal Response to Housing Needs of Older Americans, pt. 13, p. 962.

48. National Center for Housing Management, Housing for Elderly, chap. 9, p. 4.

49. Donahue, in Adequacy of Federal Response to Housing Needs
of Older Americans, pt. 13, p. 898.

50. "Medical Externship Report by the Richmond Redevelopment
and Housing Authority and Virginia Commonwealth University, Medical College of Virginia," in Adequacy of Federal Response to Housing
Needs of Older Americans, pt. 14, p. 1039.

51. Lawton, in Adequacy of Federal Response to Housing Needs
of Older Americans, pt. 14, p. 1009.

52. Carp, "Congregate Housing," p. 14.

53. Interview with James Frush, Jr., Retirement Residences,
July 26, 1976. He has developed six life-care projects in California.

54. Notte, in Adequacy of Federal Response to Housing Needs
of Older Americans, pt. 13, p. 913.

55. Lawton, in Adequacy of Federal Response to Housing Needs
of Older Americans, p. 1009.

56. Remarks by R. Michael Warren Powell, deputy minister of
housing, province of Ontario, reported in "Ontario Regional Workshop
on Housing the Elderly; Comments on Housing the Elderly and Beyond
Shelter: Proceedings," mimeographed (Ottawa: Canadian Council on
Social Development and Ontario Welfare Council, October 1974), p. 9.

57. "Letter and Enclosure from Kallia Bokser, coordinator,
Department of Social and Community Services, New York City Hous-
ing Authority," in Adequacy of Federal Response to Housing Needs of
Older Americans, pt. 14, Appendix 4, pp. 1044–45.

58. Role of the Warden in Grouped Housing (London: Age Concern, National Old People's Welfare Council, 1972).

59. "Medical Externship Report by Richmond Redevelopment
and Housing Authority and Virginia Commonwealth University, Medical College of Virginia," p. 1039.

60. Testimony by Matthew Tayback, director, Office on Aging,
state of Maryland, in Adequancy of Federal Response to Housing
Needs of Older Americans, pt. 13, p. 928.

61. U.S. Department of Housing and Urban Development, HUD
Guidelines; Lawton, Planning and Managing Housing for the Elderly.

62. Hochschild, "Disengagement Theory," pp. 553–60.

63. Testimony by Frederic Fay, Richmond (Virginia) Housing
Authority, Adequacy of Federal Response to Housing Needs of Older
Americans, pt. 14, p. 1018.

64. Lawton, Planning and Managing Housing for the Elderly,
pp. 274, 300; also Michael R. McKee and David P. McKee, "The
Elderly and Their Medical Doctors: Sociological Perspectives," un-
published paper.

65. Donahue, in Adequacy of Federal Response to Housing Needs
of Older Americans, pt. 13, p. 895.

66. Lawton, in Adequacy of Federal Response to Housing Needs of Older Americans, pt. 14, p. 1010.

67. Silverman, in Adequacy of Federal Response to Housing Needs of Older Americans, p. 990.

68. Lawton, in Adequacy of Federal Response to Housing Needs of Older Americans, pt. 14, p. 1010.

69. Carp, "Congregate Housing," pp. 15-16.

70. Testimony by Arthur H. Patterson, resident, Anthony Spallino Towers, Niagara Falls, New York, in Adequacy of Federal Response to Housing Needs of Older Americans, pt. 13, p. 920.

71. Reilly, in Adequacy of Federal Response to Housing Needs of Older Americans, pt. 14, p. 991.

72. Interview with James Frush, Jr., Retirement Residences, July 24, 1976.

73. Silverman, in Adequacy of Federal Response to Housing Needs of Older Americans, p. 990.

74. U.S. Administration on Aging, "Financing Services: Federal Resources; a Description of Title III and Title VII of the Older Americans Act of 1965, As Amended" (paper presented at the National Conference on Congregate Housing for Older People, Washington, D.C., November 11-12, 1975).

75. Silverman, in Adequacy of Federal Response to Housing Needs of Older Americans, pt. 14, p. 995.

76. Bokser, in Adequacy of Federal Response to Housing Needs of Older Americans, pt. 14, p. 1046.

77. Remarks of Senator Harrison Williams, Adequacy of Federal Response to Housing Needs of Older Americans, pt. 14, p. 990.

78. Patterson, in Adequacy of Federal Response to Housing Needs of Older Americans, pp. 920-21.

79. "Park View Plaza, Burwell, Nebraska," in Adequacy of Federal Response to Housing Needs of Older Americans, Appendix 6, pt. 13, p. 980.

80. Caroline van Mason, "Relative Costs in Food Service Programs" (paper presented at National Conference on Congregate Housing for Older People, Washington, D.C., November 11-12, 1975).

81. Thompson, "Congregate Housing for Older Adults," p. 10.

82. Lawton, Planning and Managing Housing for the Elderly, p. 309.

83. Ibid.

84. Tayback, in Adequacy of Federal Response to Housing Needs of Older Americans, pt. 13, p. 928.

85. Thompson, "Congregate Housing for Older Adults," pp. 10-12.

86. Bokser, in Adequacy of Federal Response to Housing Needs of Older Americans, pt. 13, p. 917.

87. Tayback, in Adequacy of Federal Response to Housing Needs of Older Americans, p. 928.

88. Lawton, in Adequacy of Federal Response to Housing Needs of Older Americans, pt. 14, p. 1010; Lawton, Planning and Managing Housing for the Elderly, p. 111.

89. Ibid.

90. Patterson, in Adequacy of Federal Response to Housing Needs of Older Americans, pt. 13, p. 920.

91. Thompson, "Management of Congregate Housing."

92. "Park View Plaza, Burwell, Nebraska," in Adequacy of Federal Response to Housing Needs of Older Americans, Appendix 6, pt. 13, p. 980.

93. National Center for Housing Management, Housing for Elderly.

94. Warren in Ontario Regional Workshop on Housing the Elderly, p. 11.

95. Marie McGuire Thompson, Design of Housing for the Elderly (Washington, D.C.: National Association of Housing and Urban Redevelopment Officials, October 1972), p. 10.

96. Role of the Warden in Grouped Housing.

97. John Macey, "Housing Older Adults: Management and Training" (paper presented at National Conference on Congregate Housing for Older People, Washington, D.C., November 11-12, 1975), p. 17.

98. Lawton, Planning and Managing Housing for the Elderly.

99. U.S. Department of Housing and Urban Development, HUD Handbook, p. 14.

100. Thompson, "Congregate Housing for Older Adults," p. 11.

101. U.S. Department of Housing and Urban Development, HUD Guidelines, pp. 2-3.

102. Ibid., pp. 2-3; Thompson, "Management of Congregate Housing," p. 2.

103. Lawton, Planning and Managing Housing for the Elderly, pp. 112-13.

104. Ibid.

105. Ibid.

106. "Park View Plaza, Burwell, Nebraska," in Adequacy of Federal Response to Housing Needs of Older Americans, Appendix 6, pt. 13, p. 979.

107. Carp, "Congregate Housing," p. 15.

108. U.S. Department of Housing and Urban Development, HUD Guidelines, p. 2.

109. Lawton, Planning and Managing Housing for the Elderly, pp. 224-25.

110. Ibid., p. 281.

111. Thompson, "Management of Congregate Housing," p. 3.

112. U.S. Department of Housing and Urban Development, HUD Guidelines, p. 20.

113. National Center for Housing Management, Housing for Elderly.

114. Thompson, "Management of Congregate Housing," p. 316.

115. Lawton, Planning and Managing Housing for the Elderly, pp. 224-25.

116. Thompson, "Management of Congregate Housing," p. 5.

117. Lawton, Planning and Managing Housing for the Elderly, p. 225.

118. Thompson, "Congregate Housing for Older Adults," p. 53.

119. Lawton, Planning and Managing Housing for the Elderly, pp. 222-26.

120. Silverman, in Adequacy of Federal Response to Housing Needs of Older Americans, pt. 14, p. 995.

121. U.S. Department of Housing and Urban Development, HUD Handbook.

122. Patterson, in Adequacy of Federal Response to Housing Needs of Older Americans, pt. 13, p. 920.

123. U.S. Department of Housing and Urban Development, HUD Guidelines, p. 2.

124. Thompson, "Management of Congregate Housing," p. 12.

125. Williams, in Adequacy of Federal Response to Housing Needs of Older Americans, p. 996.

126. Silverman, in Adequacy of Federal Response to Housing Needs of Older Americans, pt. 14, p. 992.

7

DESIGN OF HOUSING
FOR THE ELDERLY

Through design, the quality of life of the elderly can be en-
hanced. Through design, the manager's life, Thompson says, can
be made a joy with few complaints and accidents and without the continuous problems caused by inept planning.[1] The importance of design features in establishing a satisfactory environment for the elderly
has been stressed by managers, housing researchers, and elderly
users themselves. In our Canadian survey of elderly these users
gave design features as some of the most important reasons for satisfaction, with layout, elevators, furnishings, and size features mentioned as causes of satisfaction. At the same time the major reason
for dissatisfaction with the development expressed by these elderly
users was poor general design, with specific mention made of poor
bedroom design, lighting, noise, and closet design as well as lack
of grab rails and alarm systems[2] (see Table 7.1).

As noted previously, the various physical problems that the elderly residents in the units will have mean that the architect must
adapt his plans to meet these special needs. Most of these elderly
will be in their seventies or older and, while their limited physical
condition varies from individual to individual, most will have limited
strength and energy; this means inability to push or grip heavy doors,
to reach high shelves, to stoop to electric outlets, or bend to low
drawers. The elderly will have trouble washing clothes or preparing
a meal without sitting, or taking showers without using grab bars or
a resting bench. Their mobility is often limited, with many walking
slowly and some using a cane or a walking aid; they therefore are unable to walk down long corridors without resting on benches or using
handrails. There may be a tendency to have dizziness or loss of
sense of balance, which again means the need for frequent rest benches
or handrails if falls are to be avoided.

TABLE 7.1

Reasons for Dissatisfaction with Development

Reason	Number*	Percent
Poor general design features (bedrooms, balconies, closets, light, noise)	133	43.9
Require more special design features for handicapped (alarm system, grab rails)	16	5.3
Need elevator	9	3.0
Prefer more privacy (single rooms and private baths)	23	7.6
Total design shortcomings	181	59.7
Need more maintenance and security staff and medical services	23	7.6
Need better physical maintenance	18	5.9
Need changes in management policies and better prepared staff to deal with residents' problems	14	4.6
Staff should prevent admission of senile residents	7	2.3
Total management and staff shortcomings	62	20.5
Need more recreation services and facilities	19	6.3
Need meal services	13	4.3
Need transportation service	11	3.6
Need more facilities (tuck shop, pay phone, hairdresser, drugstore, parking)	9	3.0
Total services and facilities shortcomings	52	17.2
Need cheaper rent	14	4.6
Prefer another location	12	4.0
Other	4	1.3
No answer or no complaints	41	13.5

*The 262 residents who responded to this question gave a total of 325 reasons for dissatisfaction.

Source: Canadian user survey.

For some elderly there is a deterioriation of vision due to the atrophy of eye muslces and to cataracts, which means inability to adjust to light intensities, to see thresholds or raised floor areas, to read small signs or small telephone numbers or thermostat numbers, or to see elevator or mailbox numbers if normal size; large-size numbers are needed. Some degree of impairment of hearing is common for the elderly, which may mean difficulty in hearing apartment doorbells, fire alarms, or telephones; loud signals are needed. This hearing problem may also mean the elderly will turn their television and radio louder to compensate for the hearing impairment, and thus thicker walls are needed between the apartments.

Many elderly have some degree of arthritis or rheumatism and they have low resistance to respiratory illnesses, such as colds and pneumonia; therefore good heating is of great importance. In the study of a nationwide group of elderly in private apartments, it was found that many elderly saw heating as the main deficiency with their apartment. *

In summary, this housing must be designed to insure the maximum of safety from falls, burns, and other accidents the elderly are prone to. Moreover, the design of the unit should be planned to decrease in every way the exertions needed to do housekeeping and carry out daily activities in the apartment.

Another problem some elderly have is memory loss or some degree of senility that means they need familiar objects or landmarks or colors to help them identify their location. Each floor should be a different color.

In addition to these problems, because a number of the aged coming to these elderly apartment developments will be single, there will also be a need to provide social interaction opportunities through design. To entice the single individual out of his or her apartment, the development must include pleasing and comfortable public facilities that are usable and inviting enough for the person to feel they are an extension of his home. This is especially needed since the elderly, due to their increased leisure time or due to their illness and physical handicaps, spend much more of their time in their apartment than the younger adult does. For this reason the apartment and the complex must have a noninstitutional appearance and have the atmosphere of a place of independent living, a secure place where the person feels he belongs and that to him represents his individual home. The development needs to be in a place that allows privacy and yet, at the same time, insures security or protection from intruders.

THE APARTMENT

Since the elderly will be using their space intensely and spending much of their time in the apartment, the unit should be as appealing as possible, with careful consideration as to the use of space. To com-

---

*Special survey of the over 1,200 elderly participating in the HUD-sponsored housing allowance experiment run by Abt Associates in eight cities.

bat the feeling of closeness, this small unit needs a view to the outside world and a cheerful atmosphere, instead of a small, four-walls
cubicle feeling that can increase loneliness and depression, especially
for singles.

Size is dictated both by this intense use and financial factors;
the size problem is especially serious for singles. HUD has recommended in its Minimum Property Standards for Housing for the Elderly that there should be at least 255 square feet for an efficiency
apartment (kitchenette and dining-living-sleeping combination area)
and at least 350 square feet for a one-bedroom apartment (plus closets
and bathroom).[3] These dimensions are considered rather small by
many experts in the field.

The 1970 Canadian government publication on design for housing
the elderly also recommended a typical floor plan.[4] Architects A.
W. Cluff and P. J. Cluff, commenting in detail on these floor plans,
felt the bedroom measurements should be expanded to 12 feet 6 inches
x 9 feet 9 inches, to accommodate twin beds.[5]

In a number of developments it is felt that it is too expensive
to provide single elderly with one-bedroom units. If the unit instead
is a studio or efficiency apartment, it should be an enlarged living
room that serves as living and sleeping room. In many cases an alcove area, as in an L-shaped unit, can provide the sleeping area; in
such instances it is good if this alcove can be so placed as not to be
visible from the door so that those elderly who use the bed during
the day, due to illness, or who are more lax in their housekeeping,
will not be embarrassed by visitors seeing the unmade bed from the
door. It is not a good idea to have a hideaway bed as this is hard for
the elderly to handle.

Living Room

The living room should be so designed that there are uninter-
rupted or unbreakable areas for furniture and, if necessary, for the
bed, instead of many cut-up areas. Many elderly will bring large
pieces of furniture requiring a large area.

In every case possible, the living room windows should be large
enough to provide light and sunshine and a view; the window frames
should not have such high sills as to obscure the view when sitting.
However, where floor-to-ceiling windows or balcony doors are used,
markings should be made on them to avoid accidents. Floor-to-ceiling windows may suffer from disadvantages of extra cost in heating
and draping; they may be continually closed to sunlight by those who
desire privacy.

Old people, especially single elderly persons, like to look out.
Views of activities on a busy street may prove of special interest to

the elderly who want to passively watch what is happening in the outside world. In one Berkeley, California, development, residents
preferred the street-side apartments, with the views to a busy area,
to the apartments facing the quiet inner garden court. [6] At an Oakland,
California, complex, many of the residents spent a good part of their
waking hours close to the windows looking out on a busy business
district. Thompson complains that many architects misjudge on this
and thus design for views that are quiet, "depriving residents of the
opportunity to watch neighborhood happenings even though we know
that observation of activity is essential as participation in it decreases
and that—at best—limitations on life space are inherent in the aging
process and should be resisted. "[7]

As alternatives to the view of a busy street, planned active areas
or views can be orchestrated as part of the landscape. A Dutch elderly apartment complex in Zeist, Holland, faced a wooded park with
tame deer and ducks. In an Amsterdam development the elderly had
large garden plots right outside their window. Thompson reports that
in a French development she visited, there was a miniature zoo in the
adjacent park, cared for by the local zoo.

Walls in the apartment should be in cheerful colors. Lighting
should be good, with wall outlets at least three feet from the floor.
One should never have to walk through a dark hall to a light. If there
is a ceiling light it should not be one requiring bulb changes, as elderly should not try to reach up to change these; it should instead
have wall light fixtures. Built-in lights are the best idea.

Kitchen

The kitchen may be a full-fledged kitchen or an open galley af-
fair, as often found in a studio or efficiency apartment for a single
person. Some experts feel that an open galley kitchen is much less
preferable because of space limitations and the relegation of food
smells to the small living room area, and because some elderly,
with increased difficulty in cooking and doing housework, may have a
less than spic-and-span kitchen and be bothered if such is continually
exposed to view.

The separate kitchen may also include an eating area or alcove,
making it easier for the elderly to carry food to the table. If possible,
such an area should be near a window or living room entrance.

Kitchen fixtures such as a stove, refrigerator, and sink should
be carefully considered to be sure the limitations of the elderly are
taken into account. Regarding the stove, Thompson suggests

Front opening oven doors and controls at the back of the
stove are hazards and small numbers on the controls

make life miserable for the dim of sight and impossible
for the blind. Large numbers at the front are important.
There is rarely a light at the stove. [8]

Stove burners that have the least chance of causing fire, if left on for
a long time, should also be given priority as the absent-minded elderly person may leave the stove on. A better solution is a master
cutoff switch and an electric pilot light to show the stove is still on.

If the stove design is to be such as to avoid danger of burns,
not only should the burner controls be up front to avoid reaching over
hot burners but also all doors should have adequate clearance. The
stove should not be in a corner where the weaker left hand must be
used. Cabinets over the stove should be avoided as they are particularly hazardous. Thompson says that "the little space [around the
stove] could be better used for ventilation . . . [and] a shelf reach
of 63 inches should be maximum. Board up the rest of the space and
avoid untold broken bones and deaths from chair climbing."[9]

Regarding the sink, Cluff and Cluff[10] feel the sink should not be
in a corner; they suggest a double sink to allow laundering and suggest the faucets have large easy-to-use handles. Thompson recom-
mends the sink have space under it to accommodate a wheelchair.

One suggestion regarding the refrigerator is that it have an adequate frozen food area to allow storage of a number of days' supplies,
so that the elderly need not go out to shop in bad weather or when they
are ill.

Placement of storage space can be a problem, Cluff and Cluff
point out; they feel "full height storage is often provided at the expense
of adequate counter space and should be reconsidered. It is important
to avoid excessive reaching and stooping as many of the aged lose
their sense of balance or become dizzy, and this is extremely dangerous
in the kitchen. Direct vision of the object to be taken from the shelf
is desirable; however, this does not prevent the use of properly designed over-counter storage."[11]

Bathroom

Since the bathroom can be a place of accidents, such as slips
and falls on slippery surfaces, safety features are very important.
Grab bars by the toilet as well as in the shower or bath may be useful. An emergency bell or buzzer is now found in many bathrooms,
and when pushed sets off an alarm, sounds in the manager's apartment,
and may even unlock the front door of the apartment. Such a bell or
buzzer is an essential fixture in any apartment occupied by the elderly.
Bathroom doors should open out to allow someone to get the person
out in case of an accident.

Bathrooms should not be so small that crowded space with objects protruding menaces the elderly's movement. This is especially necessary in the case of wheelchair residents.

Placement of the toilet between the bath or shower and the basin can also help the elderly as the toilet then can be used as a seat for resting when washing clothes, shaving, or brushing teeth.

Safety versus tradition dictates whether there should be a shower or bath. There is no question many older people like and are more used to a bath; but it may be hard for many to get in or out of a bath, and such inability to negotiate the tub or, in the case of dizziness or an accident in the tub, to get out of the tub, may be a cause for continual need for staff assistance in bathing or even the cause of a move out of the development.

Talking of this debate, Lawton says:

It would be quite impossible to resolve the issue by trying to please the majority by building only one or the other [bath or shower]. In terms of safety, both a bathtub and shower entail some risk. The tub is perhaps less safe, since in addition to the risk of slipping in either shower or tub, the latter compels one to step in and out with the body precariously balanced. Some improvement is gained by making the tub height lower, and providing low and shoulder-height grab bars, plus a non-skid surface. The excessively smooth pressed-steel tubs should be avoided, and water temperature controls are mandatory. Many designers recommend strongly the shower be made with flexible tubing so that it may be used either in a high fixed position as an ordinary shower or as a shower applied locally to the body by hand. In the latter arrangement it may be used either while sitting in the tub, while standing, or while sitting on a shelf with one's legs in the tub. The sitting-position shower has much to recommend it, but requires expert human engineering to make the shelf accessible, not slippery, and near enough to the water controls to allow adjustment from the seated position. There is still considerable hazard involved in getting in and out of such a seat. [12]

Cluff and Cluff, in discussing this issue of a shower versus tub, point out that "perhaps further consideration should be given to the widely accepted fact that the elderly prefer a bath to a shower. Recent studies have suggested the contrary, that in the older age group those that have had the opportunity to experience the use of safe shower installation prefer this over the traditional bath."[13]

Thompson is stronger in her feelings about the advantages of showers:

> Universally seen are bath tubs with showers over them—
> the most hazardous of bathing arrangements. Occasion-
> ally seen is the properly designed shower with a seat,
> without curb, with a footrest flush to the wall when not in
> use, with mixed hot and cold water flowing to a testing
> spout, with tempered glass doors. [14]

She adds that "given the proper kind of shower, we may be prolonging the opportunity for the older and handicapped people to take care of themselves and yet enjoy refreshing bath without attendant."[15] We would add that if the bath is used, it should have nonskid strips, just as all the floor should be of a nonskid material and the rugs have non-skid backing. Water temperature controls should mix cold and hot water to eliminate the problem of scalding water.

The bathroom situation presents added problems in congregate housing. First, in many congregate developments, with their hotel-type rooms, expenses are kept down by having rooms share a bathroom. Second, baths and shower rooms may be at the end of the corridor. In our interviews with many residents in congregate housing a major reason for dissatisfaction with the development expressed by those who shared the bath-shower or the toilet or both was this sharing. Of those in congregate developments, a large proportion shared either bath-shower or toilet or both; in the manager survey it was reported 70 percent did. The residents complained that this sharing was inconvenient for elderly people with health problems and sudden and sometimes prolonged bathroom needs. In a Powell River, British Columbia, congregate development, many female residents shared a bathroom at the end of the hall that was very inconvenient.[16] In a Minnesota development two rooms, with two persons in each room, shared a toilet, with a door on each side, and thus their privacy was occasionally embarrassingly invaded; sometimes they left the door locked after leaving the bathroom, thus leaving the other room's occupants without access. Since both privacy and accessibility to a bathroom are needed by the elderly, we would suggest that the cost of a bathroom per room, with both toilet and shower, be given high priority. If a corridor bath-shower room is used, it should be placed midway down the hall and not at the end.

Another focus in design should be the basic bathroom-bedroom relationship, especially the distance between the two, due to the number of falls that occur between these two rooms, especially during the night. A night light should be installed so that the elderly do not stumble on the way to the bathroom at night, and a handrail put in this bedroom-bathroom corridor.

Bedroom

The bedroom may be the constant resting place of sicker residents or those returning from the hospital, and thus should not be too small and be a cheerful room, hopefully with a window and view. Moreover, since the resident has the potential of being sick for a long time, the bed should be placed where its position can occasionally be moved. The bed should not be in a corner where the elderly have trouble bending and stooping to make it. The bedroom should be large enough to have room for a television set. For a couple, the bedroom should have room for twin beds.

The apartment should have a reliable heating system that can equally penetrate all areas of the apartment. Window ventilation should be planned to avoid drafts as the elderly are especially susceptible to colds.

The apartment should have such security features as peepholes at the entrance door as well as locks that are easy to operate, yet do not automatically lock. The apartment should have phone connections in both the bedroom and the living room so that the elderly do not have to get to the living room to report a nighttime emergency or report suspicious sounds.

Apartment entrance doors should be light to the touch and there should be a loud doorbell for the hard of hearing. All the doors in the apartment should be designed for wheelchair carriers as the resident at any time may become immobilized and have to use one. A number of elderly in our Canadian developments came to the complex because they were in wheelchairs.

DESIGN FEATURES FOR PUBLIC SPACE IN
ELDERLY DEVELOPMENT

Lobby

The lobby is the most frequently used space. In some developments it is a small uninviting area, often with formal furniture no one sits in. In some developments the lobby is cheerful and inviting, a warm comfortable environment where residents sit and where the action is.

The design of the lobby may relate to its functions. Will it be one of the main sitting areas, or will there be an adjacent lounge? Will this be where the mailboxes are? Will the management office be located off the lobby? Even where a separate lounge, mailbox area, and/or office area exists, most would agree they should be so designed to be an extension of the lobby, so that people will feel they are accessible and those passing through the lobby will see it as an activity area.

The lobby should have rest benches and comfortable, inviting chairs; it should be cheerful looking with bright colors, good lighting, plants, and a bulletin board. All this will encourage use. The elderly will benefit from this since it will be an incentive for them to get out of their room. It will also help management with its security problem, especially in inner city developments, for the presence of elderly sitters in the lobby will discourage intruders. These elderly will recognize strangers to the development. If there is a receptionist or if the management office is placed in the lobby area, this double surveillance of the entrance can be quite effective. A receptionist may be necessary in inner city developments where security has become the paramount problem. For example, in one San Francisco inner city elderly housing project, located near the Tenderloin district, there have been muggings, robberies, and even one fatal attack by intruders. Residents have called numerous meetings with the housing authority to demand security guard protection and other measures to increase the safety of the residents. In some developments staff walk the elderly to and from the bus stop.

In many developments it is necessary to design the lobby in a way that limits access to strangers and limits the number of entrances, as well as eliminates dark corners, unobservable stairways, and other hiding places. The elevator area should be visible from the lobby and reception desk or windowed office. The lobby and area outside the lobby should be well lit.

The entrance to the lobby from the outside should have automatic or counterbalanced doors to make easy access possible for those elderly with limited strength or walking problems. The outside entranceway should have an overhanging drive-in area to protect the residents from bad weather while waiting for a taxi, relatives, or a bus.

Lounge

The design of other public areas should be carefully considered in terms of inviting use by the elderly. One of these is the lounge. All too often the lounge, and the lobby as well, is an area of formal, uncomfortable furniture, an area that the staff discourage residents from using, as we found in a number of Canadian elderly developments. The lounge should not be reserved for Sunday visits of relatives, Sunday services, and occasional special events. Daily use should be encouraged. It should have large windows and a pleasant view of green-

ery or street action. In one Minnesota development there was even
a bird feeding box outside one lounge window.

The lounge, like the lobby, should have comfortable chairs,
arranged in groups to enhance social interaction. The lounge should
be designed for a number of different purposes. As Lawton points
out,[17] it may be better to have low barriers or dividers that can be
put up to set off an area for a special use at the time of that event,
yet not entirely cut off other uses, thus possibly making the activity
more inviting and less isolated from other activities; he does not see
the need for a special room for each different use in all cases. Other
experts would urge that some special activities require a special
room. Some casual ones, such as card playing, may just require a
special area of the room. In the case of television watching it may
be that a special room is needed; however, one must warn that we
found in some Canadian developments that the use of the public television area was low, as most had their own television set in their
room or disliked the squabbles over program selection in the public
television room. Some activities, such as arts and crafts, may require a special room because then such supplies as a weaving loom
or paints can be stored there. A library might better be in a special
room because it assures a quiet atmosphere, but at the same time it
can be in a far corner of the lounge. The same applies to religious
services (in most Catholic developments, however, there would be a
separate chapel).

Since large developments usually have several lounges, some of
these special activities can be held in these. The floor lounges or
one of the side lounges can serve as a television watching area for
the few people who do not watch in their rooms. The dining room can
also be used for special activities and events during noneating hours.

In sum, careful consideration should be given to the type of
utilization of special rooms and whether lounges or the dining room
can be used as a legitimate substitute, before one includes these
costly rooms. In a large, and in a well-financed, development the
inclusion of such, of course, may not have to be as carefully scruti-
nized.

Another issue in providing these special rooms is whether one
will have staff to run the activities in them. It is sad to note that
in some public housing projects for the elderly they had put in special
rooms but now have them closed due to lack of staff, even from a community agency, to run programs in them.[18]

Minilounge areas should be established in two heavy traffic
places in the development. One is the mailbox area where apartment
dwellers gather every morning to wait for their mail. As our study
showed, this is a major socialization area. Comfortable chairs
should be available for sitting in that area, or in an adjacent lounge or

lobby. Congregate developments serving mainly well elderly may
have such an area, but some serving marginally competent elderly
may not, and instead have the mail delivered personally to each resident. In congregate housing another area needing a minilounge with
comfortable chairs is the area adjacent to the entrance to the dining
room. Elderly will assemble there 15 minutes or more before the
lunch and dinner meal. For some it is the main socializing period
of the day.

Dining Room

The dining room area should be so designed as to contribute to
making the meal period a pleasant social experience, as for many it
is the day's main event. The layout should make areas easily accessible by wheelchair. The decor should be bright with colored walls,
flowers and plants, colorful tablecloths and chair coverings so that
the room is warm and inviting. The 1972 HUD congregate housing
guidelines recommend:

> Some elements that contribute [to making meal service a
> pleasant social experience] would be a dining room that is
> well laid out with large spaces broken into smaller units
> of space—attractive furniture, accessories and, if possi-
> ble, with a good view in relation to out-of-door activity.
> Small tables would be preferred to large tables. If feasi-
> ble, there should also be some choice in table companions,
> as well as in the menu. A section of the dining room could
> also provide between-meal or late evening snacks.[19]

Some experts go further and say there should be a number of small
dining room areas.[20] Elegant decor, such as in the Our Lady Home
in Oakland, California, can, however, counteract the negative look
of a large room, just as bright orange colors, as in our observed
Minnesota congregate development, can make the lobby and halls
more attractive and less institutional looking.

In an apartment complex the dining room may only be used for
catered noon meals, potluck dinners, and special events; then, a
full kitchen may not be needed.

Other Facilities

If a coffee bar, canteen, or full snack bar is going to be included, it should be somewhat open and welcoming and, if possible,
adjacent to the lobby or another busy area so that users can watch the

action and can sit there with visitors. A basement or out-of-the-way location is not a good idea if high use is to be encouraged. In the observed Minnesota congregate development, the coffee bar was right off the lobby and was completely open.

If there is a small grocery-drug-general store, this should also be in an accessible location. A beauty-barber shop, however, can be easily located in the basement and often is.

A public toilet and public telephone must be located near these high-utilization facilities—lobby, ounge, mailbox area, dining room, and coffee bar—so that elderly are not forced to go back to their apartments or are not continually worried that they are too far from a toilet when needed (especially those beginning to have an incontinence problem).

A laundry is another must for apartment developments and most congregate housing, unless it is congregate serving only marginally competent. Almost all developments, as in our Canadian study, have a laundry. In many apartment complexes this area is a major socialization area for residents. It therefore should have comfortable chairs and a coke or coffee machine. The laundry should be near an elevator to limit the walking distance for users carrying a heavy load, and it should be near a public toilet. In a large multistory building a laundry may be found on every floor.

Elevators are of course needed in any high-rise development, but even if the project has only two floors an elevator may be necessary. Many elderly have trouble using stairs and, of course, for those with walking aids or wheelchairs stairs are impossible. Lack of elevators causes dissatisfaction; in our user study nine persons said it was their main reason for dissatisfaction with the development; 12 persons said they had come to the development because they had too many steps in their previous building. Provision of elevators was given as a reason for satisfaction with the development by a few residents.

Since many elderly will not be accustomed to self-manned elevators, the doors should be slow closing and the elevator slow moving, with sensitive reopening mechanism; it should have large letters on floor buttons, have good ventilation, an alarm and intercommunication system, and guard rails on the sides. It should be large enough to take not only a wheelchair but also a stretcher.

If a medical office or nurse's office is included in the building, it should, like the lounges, have a cheery reception area, instead of a stern hospital look. It should not be so centrally located that the resident or visitor has the impression this is a medical or hospital facility, a place for sick people. In fact, some would suggest that for this reason it be in a separate wing or building. Sometimes this happens because the development is affiliated with a hospital or medical clinic and uses this facility.

If there is an infirmary, the sickroom look, even use of hospital beds, should be avoided. If there is a nursing wing in the development, its appearance should also be kept noninstitutional, with bright-colored walls, a lobby rather than a nursing station look to the entry area, and hotel-type rooms with regular rather than nursing beds, when possible. In fact, the nurses' station should not be prominent and the medical look, including use of white uniforms for staff, should be minimized.

A guest room is also found in some developments, to accommodate out-of-town relatives. It should be on the first floor.

Exterior Design of Buildings

Many housing developments for the elderly have won architectural awards. Since elderly like to be proud of their buildings and show their friends and relatives they are not charity homes or institutional buildings looking like the stereotype of the old-age home of the nineteenth century of the nursing home, exterior design is important. Life-care and other luxury elderly developments have put emphasis on a luxurious-looking exterior appearance so that residents will feel more like they are moving into a Hilton for elderly rather than a home for aged sick. Many Section 202 developments, as Lawton points out,[21] are highly attractive; many cost no more per unit than public housing for the elderly but have better achieved a pleasant noninstitutional look. Some public housing for the elderly has the plain nondescriptive look or even the institutional look that has always identified it as public housing. Architectural appearance was a cause of stigma in public housing that the author saw when she wrote on this in the 1960s,[22] and it is still with us in the case of some new developments. Instead of using the same material as that generally used in the neighborhood, so that these developments blend in, the public housing authorities often use a different material and a different design, so the buildings clearly stand out as public housing.

Lack of the little special details makes the housing look stark; unattractive entranceways, cinderblock or other drab materials for exterior and interior work all make the building look shabby.

On the other hand, some public housing authorities have broken out of this syndrome and produced award-winning projects with clever use of materials. *

---

*One idea suggested by Evert H. Heynneman, chief planner, San Francisco Public Housing Authority, is not to standardize so that all elderly public housing buildings look alike.

Balconies

Balconies help to produce an attractive exterior appearance. They do, however, cost money and the question is whether they are necessary or not. This may depend on the climate and likelihood of high use. Some elderly residents will want and use balconies while others will not care. One solution is to provide some, but not all, units with balconies.

Outdoor Areas

Pleasant landscaping is necessary, for residents will spend many hours looking at the view. Even downtown developments should have some landscaped areas. Garden plots should be provided for the elderly who want such.

Outside sitting areas, especially if they are protected from street traffic, are a welcome addition, as are outside activity areas. In some regions residents may enjoy outside shuffleboard, lawn bowling, or croquet, although we found many of our surveyed elderly considered these activities too strenuous.

Security is always a concern in providing outdoor areas, just as it is a problem to worry about in deciding on site location. In high-crime areas one must worry about placement of shrubbery near the entrance and about the advisability of outside sitting areas. One must also watch out that lawn areas do not become shortcuts to other streets or to playgrounds for neighborhood children. Parking lots may have to be located in a position where they provide easy and safe access to the building. At the same time the building entry from the parking lot should not be one that invites strangers to enter and encourages loitering or vandalism.

Almost a fourth of our Canadian users moved to the development to have security and safety, although this term referred to many types of security. However, 23 of them gave as their main reason for satisfaction with the development, "adequate security in the building" (see Table 7.2). This is a concern to even a greater extent in the United States, with many elderly moving out of their private home into some sort of housing with security guards because of their fear of criminal activity. Provision of security is a major concern in housing for the elderly, with the National Center for Housing Management[23] devoting one of the longest chapters of its manual on elderly housing to the "Manager and Security." The manual points out facilities that need "site hardening" or securing, and lists necessary measures; these facilities to watch include roof, basement, elevators, stairwells, halls, and fire doors. It suggests certain specifications for security in regard to doors, locks, windows, peepholes for interviewers, mailboxes, storage rooms, offices, laundry room, garage, entrance door, and fire escapes.

Such security measures and the existence of a security staff, as found in many developments, not only lower the crime rate but give the elderly a psychological feeling of safety.

Designing for Privacy

Designing for privacy is another consideration in planning a development. Elderly want to have their own personal space designated and protected from intrusion. This is especially necessary to allow the elderly to have an independent or semiindependent living style to avoid the institutional situation of the nursing home.

TABLE 7.2

Reasons for Satisfaction with Development

Resident's Reason	Number[a]	Percent[b]
Good design features (layout, balconies, furnishings, elevators, size)	63	23.2
Privacy (own bath, no one bothers me) and independence satisfactory in this housing	63	23.2
Friendly atmosphere; easy to make and/or meet friends here; people my own age	54	19.9
Convenient location	35	12.9
Adequate security in building, including buzzer	23	8.5
Health care and other services provided	21	7.7
Good staff	18	6.6
Good meals	16	5.9
Good maintenance	16	5.9
Good selection of recreation, leisure activities, gardening	15	5.5
Reasonable rent (or best value)	10	3.7
Apartment easy to maintain	5	1.8
This housing was the only option open to me	5	1.8
No reasons given	17	6.3

[a]Some residents gave more than one reason for satisfaction.
[b]Based on the 272 residents who gave reasons they were satisfied.

Source: Canadian user survey.

It is obviously easier to achieve this in an apartment complex, where one only has to worry about the few public areas, than in a congregate housing, where there is heavy group use of many areas. Sharing of various facilities is a major hindrance to privacy. A larger proportion of our congregate development residents had to share a room and usually a bathroom and hall shower-bath facility. Many were not happy about this. Lack of privacy was a reason for dissatisfaction with the development. Yet when specifically asked about satisfaction with privacy, even 87 percent of surveyed residents in congregate and mixed developments were "very satisfied"; 91 percent in apartments were "very satisfied." Ten persons (5 percent) in congregate were "unsatisfied."

In sum, all these design features must be taken into consideration if the development is to fulfill its purpose. If there are design shortcomings, they can be major management problems, as 20 of our surveyed managers said. To the elderly, design features are important, with 21 percent of surveyed users giving good design features as their unsolicited reason for being satisfied with the development, and 49 percent in a separate open-ended question naming design features as major reasons for dissatisfaction with the development.

NOTES

1. Marie McGuire Thompson, Design of Housing for the Elderly (Washington, D.C.: National Association of Housing and Urban Redevelopment Officials, October 1972), pp. 1-2.

2. Michael Audain and Elizabeth Huttman, Beyond Shelter: A Study of NHA-Financed Housing for the Elderly (Ottawa: Canadian Council on Social Development, 1973), pp. 367-69.

3. U.S. Department of Housing and Urban Development, Minimum Property Standard (Elderly Housing), General Revision No. E-3 HUD (Washington, D.C.: Government Printing Office, 1972), p. 46.

4. Government of Canada, Central Mortgage and Housing Corporation, Housing the Elderly (Ottawa: CMHC, 1970).

5. A. W. Cluff and P. J. Cluff, "Design for the Elderly," The Canadian Architect, September 1970, p. 39.

6. Interview with Lucy Bookbinder, who, as a specialist on the elderly, was involved in planning Harriet Tubman Hall in Berkely, October 1975.

7. Thompson, Design of Housing for the Elderly, p. 5.

8. Ibid., p. 12.

9. Ibid., p. 13.

10. Cluff and Cluff, "Design for the Elderly," p. 39.

11. Ibid., pp. 39-41.

12. M. Powell Lawton, Planning and Managing Housing for the Elderly (New York: John Wiley and Sons, 1975), pp. 147-48.

13. Cluff and Cluff, "Design for the Elderly," p. 39.

14. Thompson, Design of Housing for the Elderly, p. 14.

15. Ibid.

16. Audain and Huttman, Beyond Shelter, p. 292.

17. Lawton, Planning and Managing Housing for the Elderly, pp. 165-75.

18. Testimony by Louis Danzig and Robert Notte, in Adequacy of Federal Response to Housing Needs of Older Americans, Hearings, U.S. Congress, Senate, Special Committee on Aging, pt. 13, pp. 909-13.

19. U.S. Department of Housing and Urban Development, Management of Congregate Housing: HUD Guidelines (Washington, D.C.: Government Printing Office, 1972), p. 9.

20. Marie McGuire Thompson, "Congregate Housing for Older Adults: A Working Paper" (presented to U.S. Congress, Senate, Special Committee on Aging, 94th Cong., 1st sess., 1975), p. 25.

21. Lawton, Planning and Managing Housing for the Elderly, p. 177.

22. Elizabeth Huttman, "Stigma and Public Housing: International Comparisons" (Ph.D. diss., University of California, Berkeley, 1969).

23. National Center for Housing Management, Housing for Elderly: The On-Site Housing Manager's Resource Book (Washington, D.C.: National Center for Housing Management, 1974), chap. 8.

8

SPECIAL ISSUES IN
HOUSING THE ELDERLY

ALTERNATIVE SOURCES FOR SERVICES:
DEVELOPMENT PROVISION VERSUS
COMMUNITY PROVISION

The question of whether the development itself or the community should provide the service is still an open one. There are a number of variables that must be taken into consideration in making a decision on a particular service or for a particular development. If financial considerations were of no concern, most development managers might feel they should provide a number of services, as is done in luxury life-care developments; however, in subsidized housing where expenses must be kept down, careful thought must be given as to whether the community can provide some of these services, thus saving the development money.

Various experts have considered this issue. A 1974 HUD handbook on public housing designated some services as coming from the community and others as tenant- or development-supplied services.[1] In the 1972 HUD guidelines for congregate housing, use of community is mentioned but development services and staff are emphasized.[2] Thompson and Lawton in their writings[3] both stress use of community services to cover a number of needs but they mention the use of development services, at least to meet some needs, especially when they are talking about congregate developments.

There are of course advantages and disadvantages of using either community or development sources, and it is these we explore in this section.

First, one must point out that the answer may vary according to the health of the majority of the residents of the development. The answer may vary according to whether it is congregate housing for more impaired elderly or an apartment development for mainly well elderly. The response may be based on how many elderly need the service. The response may vary according to the size of the development.

The answer may also vary by service. Some services are much more suitably supplied in the development, either because it is impractical for tenants to go outside the development for a particular service or because the service can so easily and cheaply be supplied; possibly, not much staff is needed or staff can easily be recruited, such as tenants to run certain recreational activities. In other cases, the development may have to depend on the community because the staff, such as doctors, are not easily available and are costly.

The answer as to whether the development provides the services may also relate to whether the residents demand the services in the development and can pay for them. In middle-class congregate developments both these conditions exist; sophisticated, urbane middle-class elderly are used to having housekeeping help and to having recreational services available to them. As a leading developer of life-care facilities says, what these elderly are buying is not the housing (many came from better housing) but the services.[4] In contrast, many lower-income elderly have not had services in the past and do not demand such; they are simply glad to get subsidized housing. (This does not mean they do not need the services.)

Cost, of course, is always a main reason why a development may not provide services. There is a concern that the only way one can provide services is to select tenants with the ability to pay high rents and leave out low income, a situation many hate to resort to. For example, a Richmond Redevelopment and Housing Authority official said at Senate hearings: "For congregate housing to be successful one needs facilities and services so one either needs to charge higher rents or have other agencies pay for these things."[5]

Thompson explained at Senate hearings why congregate housing has not been built:

> The first and primary reason, I believe, is the possible gap between the cost of food and other services, as well as rent, and the paying ability of very low income older persons. The [1970] Housing Act permits as an admissible expense the construction cost of a central kitchen and dining room and the necessary equipment, but the rent, food and service cost must be paid by the tenants. LHA's can plainly see the result of this gap. It means that they could only select for residence those elderly persons who could defray total costs. . . . This is an unwelcome departure from the traditional and more humane tenant

selection process of selecting by need, and the more minimal the income, the greater the need. . . . The services
cost gap has been a most effective barrier to the development of congregate housing by local housing authorities.[6]

Thompson, arguing for a HUD subsidy to allow the development
to contract for services and staff, adds:

Subsidy commitment might be further controlled by requiring that to the degree possible, and for as long as possible,
those services that exist in the community for which any
low income elderly person is eligible, should first be called
upon on behalf of the tenants of congregate housing.[7]

The ironic aspect of this very serious cost consideration is that, first,
whether the community supplies the service or the development is
allowed to have a subsidy, cost comes out of federal coffers, in some
cases the same program budget. Second, costs for a subsidy for services to elderly housing complexes can be so phenomenally lower than
the cost now incurred to keep these same impaired elderly in a nursing home under Medicaid, that to deny such a subsidy seems illogical.
Quite rightly, the director of the state of Maryland Office on Aging, in
budgeting for subsidization of service costs for elderly housing, said
the reason was that "a major definite consideration is the offset gained
in leveling off and minimizing payments in Medicaid for nursing home
care."[8] He estimated that in public housing converted to congregate
housing, the cost of food, the cost of housekeeping assistance, and
the cost of general supervision, all in this package, would add $150
to $200 a month on to the cost of the housing in 1975.
      Under these circumstances, many insist that only the community
can provide most services (except meals in the congregate units);
the development cannot afford to if it is to charge reasonable rents.
While there are a variety of reasons why this is advantageous, there
are also compelling reasons why it does not always work or prove
suitable.

Advantages of Community Provision of Services

One main advantage of community provision of services is that
the community has a better chance to get a federally funded program
such as information and referral, recreational programs, homemaker
services, or transportation services, under Title III of the Older
Americans Act or Title XX of the Social Security Act, or other federal or state programs. (At the same time HUD has an agreement

with HEW whereby some of this funding should go directly to the development, as mentioned elsewhere.)

Even the AOA Title VII nutrition-meals program may be more likely to go to a neighborhood senior citizen center than to an elderly apartment development, as Bokser of New York City Housing Authority[9] has pointed out; some area office on aging people feel public housing staff are not socially oriented enough to take on this job, and they feel public housing elderly are already a privileged elderly group, compared to the private elderly renter.

A second advantage is that the community, catering to all the elderly in the area, can provide a wider array of services than the development can with possibly professional staff, more staff, and better facilities. This comparison would be especially true if the development were a small one. In a small development only a few people might need the service.

A development can benefit from community services by setting up a special relationship, say, with a hospital or medical clinic it is near or affiliated with, or a church organization social center of the same religious affiliation. A development might especially be inclined to depend on community services if it is in a downtown location near many of these services.

Another major reason for using community services is that it gets the elderly out of the development, makes them travel about the community and be more active, and mixes them with nondevelopment elderly. It thus avoids the stagnation and segregation that can occur if the development residents do not get out into the community. Such stagnation is especially deadly in small developments where there are few people to mix with, a situation our surveyed elderly complained about. Unfortunately in this Canadian user survey, too few (less than half) of these elderly said they got out one hour or more daily and they definitely participated less in community organizations than they had before they came to the development; before coming to the development almost half (46 percent) had participated weekly or monthly in community activities, and after coming to the development only slightly over a fourth did (28 percent).

Use of community services, however, has disadvantages. In our research a complaint about visiting nurses was, first, that they missed some cases that needed assistance but did not come to them; second, they were not able to give enough long-term attention to the same cases to really be of help. Another complaint was that their visits were infrequent and they were not available on weekends when medical emergencies often occurred. These same complaints can apply to services other than nursing.

Another disadvantage already mentioned is that social agencies, feeling the development residents are already privileged and helped, might feel the agency's resources are needed more to help community elderly. These agencies, especially if nonprofit, often have very limited budgets. They may feel if they service this concentrated group of elderly, they will have little time and money left to serve the dispersed community elderly. One nonprofit agency providing services to one of our surveyed developments actually found itself in this situation. Another problem the development faces in using community services is that the agency very likely will not be able to make a long-term commitment to supply the services because it cannot predict its own long-term financial resources and direction of provision. Thompson considered this a problem for congregate developments needing services. She said, regarding the problem of agency annual appropriations in relation to long-term needs of congregate developments:

> As a minimum, it requires about eighteen months to acquire land, design and construct housing. While service agencies may make a moral commitment for the services component, they would not be able to guarantee either the availability of funds in a second year of appropriations, nor could they guarantee their continuation.[10]

Another problem with use of community services is that if they are ones that do not normally serve the elderly, they may not understand the special needs and problems this group has. Moreover, having stereotypes of the elderly, they might not even want them as clientele, as is true with some doctors.

Another disadvantage is that the development elderly do not feel welcome in some community agencies and thus may not use the service. For example, some in our user survey who did not use a community senior citizen center mentioned, as one reason among several, that they "don't like the people there." They also mentioned "it was hard to get to." This could relate to the development being isolated, in an inaccessible outer area. If the development is so located, it will be hard to depend on community services.

If many of the residents have health limitations that make it hard for them to get around, then, unless a minibus or other transportation is provided, they may not be able to use community services. For example, a fifth of our surveyed elderly used a cane, crutch, brace, or artificial limb, and 3 percent had special shoes and another 3 percent a wheelchair or walker. Almost a third had difficulty getting places and 7 percent did not go out; the total in these two categories was only 26 percent for apartment residents but 43 percent for congregate and mixed developments. Thus it is hard for this part of the group to get to community services.

If a community service is used, a development staff member must see that transportation is available for some residents; he must see that the elderly know the hours and days the community service is open, or, in the case of medical services and social work or legal counseling, have an appointment made for the elderly user. The staff member must establish rapport with these agencies, pass on necessary facts about users, and see that these development elderly get good treatment. Last, the staff must take on the advocacy job of finding those elderly in need in the development and seeing they get to services.

Advantages of Using Development Services

A major advantage of using development services is that one is bringing services to those elderly in the development who have mobility problems or for other reasons do not go out into the community, especially in the winter in northern areas. If it is a meal service, say, one meal a day for apartment dwellers, this would be especially true. Second, with development services one has more chance of getting those reluctant to use the service to participate, whether they be withdrawn and isolated elderly or the passive introvert types. Advocacy tactics can work better if one only has to encourage nonusers in need of a service to go downstairs to the service rather than across town for it. If the development is isolated, this especially applies.

Another advantage is that if the service is in the development, obviously the staff has more control over the service, can shape it to their needs, and staff it as they see fit. The management can make sure it meets the specific needs of their elderly residents and that there is a follow-through of long-term help for the needy person. One can also make sure the service is not erratic or is not simply a minimal, almost dormant service.

If the development provides certain services, it means it will have to have facilities for these, and sometimes these facilities can be used for a number of services and special events. (Unfortunately, the reverse has happened as well, that is, the public housing development has the facility but has no funds to run it and so must close the facility.)[11]

Likewise, if the development can get funds for a service, such as those under Title III of the Older Americans Act or Title XX of the Social Security Act, or even funds for the AOA meals program under Title VII of the Older Americans Act, they may get some other services, such as information and referral or recreation services, as spinoffs, as well as get special staff. It may also allow them to use residents as staff, as is true for many Title VII meal programs.

Sometimes the development can get the service free because an affiliate comes in and provides it, such as a religious group or an ethnic organization, as in the Jewish homes for the aged or, for example, the Finnish-Canadian organization in Vancouver; in the latter case they not only provide religious services and recreational programs, but special dinners and sometimes social counseling. In another case the family service agency provided the service.

Another advantage to the development having these services in the development, including those provided by the above organizations, is that it helps give the development a friendly air. And, because there are services such as recreational activities or meals, residents have more chances for contact with each other. In our user survey, where the services were in the development the residents seemed more satisfied with the development.

Disadvantages to Provision by Development

One disadvantage, already mentioned, is the high cost to the development both of providing the service and providing the facility; especially in a small development, one might not have enough users for many services. Also, the services may duplicate some already existing in the community, which, in the case of a downtown development, may be quite nearby.

Another disadvantage already mentioned is that tenants get stagnated when they do not have chances to meet community elderly or participate in community activities. The more that services are provided in the development, the less likely they are to get out.

Provision of these services, some say, will also introduce premature dependency.[12] Another complaint is that if medical services are provided, it creates a "sickness" atmosphere in the development that very healthy elderly do not want to associate with, as it puts them, they feel, in a grouping they are not ready for.

Well elderly also may not choose to come to a development that serves meals or has compulsory housekeeping because they do not want to pay for a service they do not yet need, and they want the independence and privacy of an apartment development. Others, who do need the services offered more in congregate housing, may not come just because they cannot afford the higher monthly rent of congregate housing.

Another aspect of the development supplying the services is that for some federal funding, the service must also be offered to outsiders. Such a policy is approved not only by U.S. housing and geriatric experts but European experts. Ernest Noam mentions in his book on European elderly housing the degree to which developments hold themselves responsible for placing their social and health facilities at the disposal of other elderly persons living nearby and serving them by providing a senior center. He says:

> Scandinavian countries are advanced in developing institutions which are accessible to older persons outside. The elderly from the surrounding community can pass the entire day in the home or its affiliated club, and they can utilize cultural activities, occupational therapy, and physical therapy at these facilities. A dining room or restaurant is at their disposal. This opening out into the outside world also provides residents with new personal contacts and an interest in outside affairs. [13]

Community-Development Service

Many experts recommend having a service for all in the community provided in a development facility because it breaks down the wall between residents and elderly outsiders, decreases the segregation of the development from the community. A number of senior citizen centers have been put in the developments; Title VII noon meal programs for the neighborhood have been put in elderly housing complexes. Nursing services for the neighborhood are sometimes in development facilities. Day care centers for the elderly have been suggested for or exist in elderly developments, though more likely as a wing of a nursing home. Religious services for both community members (possibly of a particular ethnic group) and residents are found in a number of developments. The New York City Housing Authority was among the first to pioneer in providing facilities and through its community service division encouraging agencies to come in and use them to provide services to the neighborhood and tenants.

The major problem with a community service in a development facility is that the residents consider it their service and make outsiders feel unwelcome and feel residents dominate the service. We found this in several developments. If it is a day care facility, residents may resent sicker elderly using their development. [14] If both residents and outsiders should use the service, it is best if they are of similar socioeconomic background. [15]

Whether the arrangement used, then, is one of community services or provision of community services in the development, or provision of development services for residents only, there are advantages and disadvantages. One must take into account the many variables mentioned above.

MULTILEVEL CARE COMPLEXES FOR
THE ELDERLY

Another issue in housing the elderly concerns whether the development should be a one-level care facility, such as apartments
for well elderly, or a multilevel care complex that includes apartments
for independent ambulatory elderly, congregate housing for somewhat
impaired elderly, and a nursing home facility for elderly with serious
health problems.

In these discussions the real issue is whether the nursing wing
should be included, as many developments have both the apartment
and congregate housing and this is generally accepted. This type of
combination is likely to become more popular, for as residents of
apartment developments age, their health often deteriorates and they
have need for more services. Public housing authorities, faced with
an aging population, are talking more of providing congregate wings to
take care of this crisis situation. About 10 percent of the surveyed
developments of the 294 in our manager study were mixed developments, having both an apartment and congregate wing. Some nonprofit
ones, especially those run by religious orders, also had a nursing
wing, often with nuns as nurses. But in general a nursing wing is
only found in middle-class Section 231 developments or entirely private developments. Luxury life-care developments usually have a
nursing care or long-term care-convalescence wing; in fact they have
such as a major feature that insures lifetime security for the residents.[16]

Some developments have a wing that is somewhere in between
congregate housing and a nursing home; they have personal care staff
and one or two RNs but they do not take the serious nonambulatory
patient found in many nursing homes. Most would not take anyone
who could harm others or himself. Such a development may be a congregate development that has an infirmary; when a few residents become too impaired for the other wings, they receive long-term care
there. If a number become quite impaired, the congregate development may set aside a more highly staffed wing for them, as done at
Powell River development, British Columbia, or it may expand its
complex to take care of these longtime residents, as is true for one
private San Francisco development.

This type of use change also is found in European homes for the
aged, as Noam reports in his book on these homes. He says this
housing is for those in good health except for minor complaints, but
he reports that many of these homes have "an infirmary . . . essentially for the treatment of acute illness, but also to enable residents
to remain in the home even after they grow older."[17] Noam also
predicts there will be more multilevel facilities in the future:

It appears that these combined [multilevel] systems will
flourish in the future. Whereas some countries, e.g.,
the German Federal Republic, prefer a system combining
service flats [apartments], old people's homes, and
nursing homes, it is generally coming to be recognized,
particularly in Scandinavian countries, that it is more
practical to construct service flats equipped with nursing
personnel in connection with nursing homes. As a rule,
centers for the elderly are affiliated with these institutions.[18]

The author observed such multilevel developments in Amsterdam
(with an official of the Amsterdam Municipal Housing Authority, in
the summer of 1971). A particularly pleasant-looking one in a new
area of Amsterdam had apartments with large glass windows; there
were beautiful garden plots in front of the windows that residents
tended themselves. The apartments had an emergency alarm system
and daily reporting system. The complex had a congregate living
wing or building next to the apartments; on the other side of that was
a modern high-rise geriatrics hospital with large windows. Residents
told the author they felt secure knowing the hospital wing was there;
a spouse could be taken to the hospital and still be near his wife,
who continued to occupy the apartment, or they both could move to
the congregate living wing. Some said they were happy to know they
could get meals in case one of them were sick.

Developments can see certain advantages to having a multilevel
facility for humanitarian reasons. It means development managers
do not have to go through the traumatic experience of asking seriously
and chronically ill elderly to leave the development. The manager is
reluctant to do this because he knows the move to the nursing home
can mean premature functional death.

Public housing authorities have seen many of their elderly residents deteriorate to the point that they must ask them to leave for
the nursing home or they must bring more services. Officials concerned with this crisis situation have been quoted above as saying a
major worry in regard to this is trying to locate nursing homes that
will take these elderly.[19]

Many nursing homes that take low-income elderly have long
waiting lists. Therefore many housing managers have no place to
send these elderly. Some keep them, and this means some apartment
developments begin to have an institutional look; the projects also
develop the appearance of underserviced areas, with elderly sitting
about, getting less assistance than they need.

Congregate developments face the same problems with elderly
who can no longer walk to the dining room, manage even the basic

personal care, or stay continent; as we said, some may be senile, have delusions, hallucinations, or depressions. Some of these cases may have a health problem that means need for an in-between stage of care, more than some congregate housing offers but less than a nursing home. Lawton reminds us of this:

> Some of these more obvious disabilities may affect only limited sectors of the individual's life: hearing difficulty, partial vision, physical disfigurement, or the necessity for cane, crutches or walker which look unpleasant to others but do not usually in themselves necessitate removal. Even where forgetfulness becomes obvious, or a decline in personal neatness occurs, extra work by the manager in listening to the complaints of offended tenants, and talking to them about helping the declining tenant may prolong his stay.[20]

Keeping such a person in the development is helped if there is a wing with more intensive care than in the normal congregate arrangement. Such a move to a more intensive care wing is not as major a decision for a manager as the move out of the development to a nursing home, does not mean dramatic conferences with the doctor and with a family. Since the family often is unable to accept the fact that their elderly parent has deteriorated to the point where he or she needs intensive nursing care, and thus cannot understand why their parent is being asked to move from the congregate or apartment housing, if an intensive care wing exists, the situation is so much more easily and less dramatically handled, both for the family and the manager. Lawton backs this up, saying "there is some reason to think that a move may be less traumatic when it involves only a change in apartments within the same building or a change from one unit of a multiservice facility to another. Thus, the administrator who has a special-care area in his building or a nursing home next door will have less reason for anxiety about the effect of the move on the tenant."[21] The administrator will not have to worry that he is sending people away to die. In one studied development the worry also was whether they were sending their elderly on to nursing homes where no one spoke their language, Finnish, or cooked their type of food. From the development's point of view another advantage of including a nursing wing is that it means the development has adequate nursing and medical staff that can be made available to all its residents in emergencies. It also means a possible cost saving, for instead of keeping elderly who develop major health problems in the congregate wing, giving them heavy staff attention (because one hates to evict them from the development), with a nursing wing available, one can move them

into that wing when more intense care is needed and in many cases
Medicaid will meet some or all costs.

Many elderly themselves would like the development to include
a nursing wing. Since many of our surveyed elderly residents had
expressed a desire for more nursing care and 24-hour surveillance-
emergency care, it is not surprising that almost three-fourths favored
a multicare accommodation with a variety of types of boarding care
and full nursing care in the same development; 35 percent "definitely"
and 37 percent "somewhat" favored it. Only 17 percent were opposed
(12 percent "somewhat" and 6 percent "definitely" opposed—see Table
8.1).

Responses, however, were a little more divided than this would
indicate, with those with physical incapacities much more likely in
favor of a development that included a full nursing care wing, and well
elderly much less likely to favor it; 87 percent of the residents with
serious limited ability were definitely in favor of multicare accommodation, compared with 30 to 32 percent of those in all the health
categories definitely in favor. However, when the responses that
"definitely" and "somewhat" favored such an accommodation were
combined, the differences between the four health categories were
not great. And only a small group in any health category "somewhat"
or "definitely" disfavored such a multicare housing complex, though
there were differences, with none of the seriously incapacitated, only
around 13 to 15 percent of the moderately and slightly incapacitated,
but 22 percent of those with no incapacity, disfavoring it. Congregate
development residents were more likely to favor the multilevel complex than were apartment dwellers. A few residents did seem to be
against a mix when they gave as a reason for dissatisfaction with the
development, "Staff should prevent admission of senile residents."

Lawton also found some resistance by some well elderly to a
complex with a special care wing, in this case in his Philadelphia
Geriatric Center's York House South elderly housing:

> It is probably true that the presence of the special care
> area screens out a certain number of people who are over-
> sensitive to the "sick" atmosphere from every applying for
> admission. We have determined that the applicants to York
> House South [with its special care area which includes 24-
> hour nursing care and is a medical operation] are older or
> less independent than those applying to some other hous-
> ing.[22]

Lawton warns that having a nursing wing can contribute to changing the total milieu in the direction of the "sick" environment:

TABLE 8.1

Opinion Concerning Value of Mixed Accommodation, by Health Status

Health Status	Response to Notion of Mixed, Self-Contained, Congregate, and Nursing Accommodation						
	Definitely Favor	Somewhat Favor	Don't Know	Somewhat Oppose	Definitely Oppose	No Answer	Total
Seriously limited ability							
Number	13	2	0	0	0	0	15
Percent	86.7	13.3	0	0	0	0	100
Moderately limited ability							
Number	16	18	11	4	4	0	53
Percent	30.2	34.0	20.8	7.5	7.5	0	100
Slightly limited ability							
Number	35	44	11	12	4	2	108
Percent	32.4	40.7	10.2	11.1	3.7	1.9	100
No incapacity							
Number	41	48	10	19	9	0	127
Percent	32.3	37.8	7.9	15.0	7.1	0	100
Total							
Number	105	112	32	35	17	2	303
Percent	34.7	37.0	10.6	11.6	5.6	0.7	100

Note: Mixed accommodation means a combination of self-contained apartments, congregate units, and a nursing unit.

Source: Canadian user survey.

A substantial <u>minority</u> of tenants would prefer not to have
such a service in the same building where they live.
Some are also very sensitive to the fact that this floor
populates the dining room with "sick"-looking people and
causes nurses in uniform to be visible in other areas of
the building. [23]

In a development we observed in Minneapolis, the top floor was
a nursing care section and the patients on this floor had to eat and interact there. Residents of the congregate part, the lower floors, did
not welcome them there, especially in the lounge. In one development
in Ottawa that had a special floor for nursing cases, residents of the
lower congregate floors expressed the fear they might be moved to
the nursing floor; one can see the fear as well as the relief of having
the wing.

Yet Lawton found, as we did, that "when questioned in depth
about their attitudes to the special-care facility, tenants frequently
could say in the same sentence that they didn't like its being located
in their building, but that it was still a good thing, a service they
themselves might need someday. For this population, at least, the
net balance was obviously in favor of having a place to go to if one's
health declined." [24] This attitude is also indicated by Carp's [25] public housing elderly sample, restudied after eight years, where a
quarter wanted more complete medical and health care services, but
nonintrusive.

Donahue, in her survey of 182 local housing authorities with
housing for elderly, [26] found 71 percent of these authorities had a preference for mixed populations in a project of fully independent and
semiindependent tenants. But these authorities seem to be talking of
a mix that would not include nursing wing residents, and they were
more concerned about having enough independent residents, or healthier ones, in the mix with semiindependent, for those supporting the
mix gave such comments as the following:

Mixed occupancy would lend itself to a much healthier living environment. Having to reside and associate with
only semi-independent residents for the remainder of one's
life would, in our opinion, tend to be very discouraging.
. . . Our preference is for a mixed population to avoid a
"nursing home connotation." . . . We prefer a mixed
tenant group—the fully independent residents could help
the less mobile by carrying food, helping with housework,
et cetera, and be paid a small fee for it. [27]

Thus these authorities seem to be saying that in congregate
they want a mix of the healthy and the less healthy, or they want a
complex including congregate housing and apartments.

Thompson's comments on mixed levels of residents in congregate housing also are addressed more to mixing residents of different
health status in one type of development:

> In some places it also may be necessary to combine in one
> development residents who need or want services with others
> who are hale and hearty with no service needs. In this
> type of mixed development, however, the hale and hearty
> should be in the majority. If the more frail or impaired
> residents were in the majority, we should expect the de-
> velopment to lose some of its appeal to the well and ac-
> tive elderly—they may not be disposed to live in an atmos-
> phere that they perceive to be one of declining abilities and
> increasing dependency. When combining older people with
> such varying levels of functional capacity in one develop-
> ment, the management should avoid two prescriptions:
> (1) the more frail or impaired or handicapped should not
> be segregated in specific locations in the building; and
> (2) the more active should not be required to use services
> intended primarily for the more frail or impaired (e.g.,
> the taking of meals). While the arrangements required in
> such mixed developments will have cost implications, they
> increase the potential of such developments to attract a
> larger proportion of the elderly who can live independently
> and desire to continue doing so.[28]

This idea of mixing well and semiindependent is controversial if it is
carried to its extreme, that is, having the fully healthy, and the
somewhat seriously impaired elderly, those who could easily qualify
for a nursing home, in the same wing; yet many congregate developments, as mentioned earlier, have a range of health types, with some
having seriously impaired elderly.

The second point here, that well elderly must be in the majority, may also be controversial. In many multilevel care complexes,
with apartment and congregate wings, well elderly are more likely
to be in the apartment part, and impaired in the congregate wing, as
this wing was included or added to house those with health limitations
and who therefore need services. Of course, as we mentioned above,
one limitation in one part of the body might not qualify them as seriously impaired elderly.

Another controversy is over whether the nursing wing should
be built when the rest of the development is built or should be added

to the development at a later date, when the residents start to age
to the point that some need nursing care. Carp[29] favors the general
idea of adding services and facilities when the need arises, and adding them in a way that meets the specific need. This add-on idea has
merit for another reason, that is, it will prevent to some degree premature use of this nursing wing because the wing will not be built
until the need is great. On the other hand, one might want to plan and
build the whole complex at one time if for no other reason than to
save building costs.

When the nursing wing is included, it should be made to look as
little like a hospital or institution as possible, with decorated halls,
apartment-like rooms with regular beds, a disguised or hidden nursing station, and a limitation on the number of staff in white uniforms.

In conclusion, there are many arguments for a multilevel facility
but some disadvantages. It is likely we will see more of it in the future.

SIZE OF THE DEVELOPMENT

Size of the elderly apartment or congregate development is an
issue on which experts differ. Those favoring small developments of
less than 75 units argue that small projects mean the elderly are dispersed and scattered throughout the community rather than concentrated.
They feel the small project is more intimate and homey.[30] The manager gets to know all the residents, and residents interact more with
each other; there is little chance for the elderly person to be isolated
or ignored.

It is also argued that it is easier for the elderly person to make
the adjustment from his or her home to a small homey project than
to a big one. The small project is less likely to take on an institutional atmosphere.

Other experts argue that the medium-size or large project need
not be bad.[31] People get to know others on their floor or in their
wing. While the manager might not know everyone, he will have an
assistant manager or social service staff who can have as part of their
job contact with the residents. The medium-size or large project
will have more services and facilities than the small development as
well as more staff. This of course will be a major benefit to the elderly. The small development cannot afford specialized staff such as
a social worker or nurse, nor will it be feasible to have a crafts
room, infirmary, or other special rooms for a small group. Lawton
suggests that "small projects should not accept people of marginal
competence unless they provide some special means to oversee their
welfare." His concern, obviously, is that there will not be the ser-

vices needed by marginally competent elderly in these small developments. [32]

It is also argued that in a small project there are seldom enough tenants interested in a particular social activity to be able to carry it on. Thus it is hard to have an active and diversified social program in a small development. Residents will have to turn more to community activities, as we found was true for residents of small projects in our Canadian survey.

Above all, it is argued that the small development is not economically feasible. Even if many facilities are left out, some are so essential that they must be included, and if their cost is divided among 20 units instead of 80 or 100 units, it is much higher. The same is true of staff. To run a good development, one will still want a manager and maintenance man, and the cost per resident in a 20-unit building is considerably more than for a 100-unit building. This situation applies even more for congregate housing than for apartment developments because it is essential in congregate housing serving impaired elderly to have the staff, the services, and the facilities. And, of course, it is hard to operate a dining room for a small group.

Because of these reasons, many agree a small development may have disadvantages. However, in the medium-size or large development every effort must be made to avoid an institutional atmosphere and a regimented living style with rules and red tape. Moreover, the staff must make every effort to seek out the isolated elderly and to create a homey atmosphere.

The findings from our Canadian research supported the idea that medium-size developments had many more services than the small developments. In our survey of 294 managers of developments, those in projects with 20 residents or less and even 40 or less said they had few services available, including voluntary transportation and voluntary friendly visiting; in addition, many of these developments had no staff and only a few of these small developments had more than two in staff. None of the very small developments (20 residents or less) had a staff and only a fourth of the developments of 21-40 residents did. Most of these small developments were in rural areas.

In our other study, of 303 elderly in 19 of these Canadian developments, we again found the small developments had fewer services than larger developments, and the elderly living in these small developments (here defined as 40 units or less) were less likely to be satisfied with the development. From 65 to 85 percent of those interviewed in each large (150 units or more) development said in general they were very satisfied with living in the development; the same was true for those in the medium-size (41-150-unit) developments. Lumping all small developments together, only 26 percent of their interviewed residents were "very satisfied." In four of the

seven small developments, the proportion of "very satisfied" was indeed lower, with only 9 to 46 percent, depending on the development,
"very satisfied"; in the other three small developments, 75 to 93
percent were "very satisfied."

When asked if their building was "too large or too small or
just right," most in the large developments felt the size was just
right, with only one or two elderly in each development responding
otherwise. However, in two large developments, a third said the development was "too large." Almost no one interviewed in any of the
medium-size developments (41-150 units) felt the development was
too large; a few felt it was too small. A few in the small developments
(40 units and under) felt the size was too small and the rest said the
size was all right.

From this data we cannot say there is a strong negative feeling
among users toward large or medium-size developments; in fact the
medium-size development seems to be the preferred one. Also,
these larger developments do have more staff and services and thus
can better serve the elderly's needs.

SITE LOCATION

Location of housing for the elderly is a major decision that will
affect the elderly's satisfaction with the housing and, in fact, their
desire and ability to stay in this type of housing. Their physical limitations, as well as lack of a car in many cases, mean a decreased
mobility; their social world and their spatial orientation will be mainly
in terms of the development and its immediate neighborhood of a
five-to-ten block radius (see Table 8.2). Their interest will be in
having this environment be a pleasant and secure one that is above all
accessible to services they need.

Downtown Versus Outer Area Location

In former days, homes for the aged, as well as mental institutions, were put in quiet, pastoral rural sites, often with large gar-
dened grounds. Favor has turned from these isolated sites to those
in more active close-in locations. HUD and other sources now recommend such. Findings from our Canadian nationwide research show
reasons to favor this location choice. European research also does.
Writing on European housing for the aged, Noam points out:

Investigations have shown that old people generally prefer
to live in or near the urban center, even though they have

TABLE 8.2

Degree of Movement Outside Development, by Type of Development and Location

Type of Development and Location	Not Daily or Irregular	Daily Less Than One Hour (and maybe less in winter)	Daily One Hour or More (except possibly winter)	No Answer	Total
All self-contained apartment developments					
Number	40	15	61	0	116
Percent	34.5	12.9	52.6	0	100
Downtown location					
Number	18	8	31	0	57
Percent	31.5	14.1	54.4	0	100
Residential location					
Number	22	7	30	0	59
Percent	37.7	11.9	50.4	0	100
All congregate and mixed developments					
Number	57	55	74	1	187
Percent	30.4	29.4	39.5	0.7	100
Downtown location					
Number	11	17	31	0	59
Percent	18.6	28.8	52.6	0	100
Residential location					
Number	46	38	43	1	128
Percent	35.9	29.7	33.5	0.9	100
Total					
Number	97	70	135	1	303
Percent	32.0	23.2	44.5	0.3	100

Source: Canadian user survey.

less garden space at their disposal. A central location provides them with more opportunities to participate in outside activities and to exchange visits among friends.[33]

Since many housing sponsors may still be undecided as to advantages of an inner area site, it is useful to give details on these findings regarding downtown versus outer area sites, especially since most elderly housing is in urban locations.

Accessibility

A major advantage of downtown sites compared to outer area sites is accessibility to services. Since this is important to elderly, it must be taken into account. In our Canadian survey of 294 managers of elderly developments, 80 percent of the downtown site managers said none of the facilities were difficult to reach; this proportion dropped to 69 percent and 69 percent for residential neighborhood and suburban development managers, respectively, and down to 55 percent in the case of rural managers. As for three or more services being difficult to get to, only 4 percent of downtown development managers said this situation existed, while 15 percent of the older residential and the suburban development managers did. In fact these downtown developments were twice as likely to be described as affording an easy walk to the shopping center as were residential or suburban area developments (85 percent versus 45 percent and 47 percent, respectively). As for accessibility by foot to the grocery store and medical center, facilities the elderly very much want near them, differences again were found between downtown developments and others, as they also were for accessibility to a senior citizen center; in all cases downtown developments were more accessible to these specific services. In general, outer area managers were likely to say it was an easy bus ride to the service while downtown developers said an easy walk. Social contact service, such as a friendly visiting service, telephone contact service, and social work counseling were also less likely to be available to outer area developments than to downtown developments (see Table 8.3).

In summary, one must conclude that data from this survey of 294 managers indicate that in Canada many developments are sited in such a way that they have accessibility problems, because a third of the 294 are in suburban areas, over a third in older residential areas, 6 percent in rural areas, and only a fourth in downtown locations. Many are described as "isolated from other residences on the street" by their manager rather than as just another residence on the street. Again suburban and rural development managers were more likely than downtown development managers to describe their building as isolated, though differences were not great.

TABLE 8.3

Evaluation of Closeness of Most Services, by Location

Location	5 of 8 Services Not Close	3–4 of 8 Not Close	2 or Less Not Close	All Close	No Answer	Total
Downtown						
Number	0	2	9	43	12	66
Percent	0.0	3.0	13.6	65.2	18.2	100
Older residential						
Number	8	4	13	55	25	105
Percent	7.6	3.8	12.4	52.4	23.8	100
Suburban						
Number	3	7	14	48	16	88
Percent	3.4	8.0	15.9	54.5	18.2	100
Rural						
Number	1	0	4	6	4	15
Percent	6.7	0.0	26.7	40.0	26.6	100
No answer						
Number	3	1	5	6	5	20
Percent	15.0	5.0	25.0	30.0	25.0	100
Total						
Number	15	14	45	158	62	294
Percent	5.1	4.8	15.3	53.7	21.1	100

Source: Canadian manager survey.

In the user survey of elderly residents in selected Canadian developments, accessibility was again highlighted as a problem by outer area development residents. In this survey almost two-thirds of the respondents lived in developments located outside downtown areas. Many in this group felt there was not easy access either by walking, bus, or car to services important to them, such as neighborhood grocery stores, shopping center, medical offices, church.

While health influenced their response, location was found to influence it even more. Healthwise, data showed 9 percent of those with no health problem said there was not easy access, and at the other extreme, three-fourths of the small group with serious limitations answered either "not easy access to services," or, more likely, "they don't go out" (three-fourths of this group—see Table 8.4). However, when health was controlled, downtown location definitely influenced the likelihood of a positive response on accessibility to services. At most of the downtown location developments in this user study, none of the elderly said the location meant inaccessibility to most or all important services; however, at two such developments a fifth said such inaccessibility existed. This meant those with health limitations as well as those with no physical incapacity found accessibility to services satisfactory. For example, at one Toronto congregate living development, three-fourths of the interviewed elderly were aged 80 or over, a third had serious or moderately serious health limitations, and one-third had difficulty getting out, yet only one person said there was not easy access to services and 46 percent got out one hour or more daily (except possibly in winter). At another downtown development, 13 percent had health limitations, and one-fifth difficulty in getting places, yet no one felt that there was not easy access to services and 71 percent got out daily (except possibly in winter).

In comparison, interviewed elderly in residential area locations complained considerably of inaccessibility and were much less likely to get out daily. Though health and age account for this to some degree, most were in no poorer health than those at the downtown Toronto development and the other downtown development mentioned above.

Over half at four of these outer area developments said there was not easy access to major services; at three of these developments residents went out very little. In fact, in all outer area congregate developments only a third of interviewed residents said they went out one hour or more daily (except possibly in winter), while in all downtown congregate developments over half (53 percent) of the residents said they went out one hour or more daily. Health differences were minor.

An outer area or downtown location also had an effect on the degree to which residents participated in community organizations.

TABLE 8.4

Access to Important Services, by Health Status

Health Status	Easy Access to Services (including if elderly drive)*	Easy Access to Some but Not All	Somewhat Easy Access	Not Easy Access	Don't Go Out	No Answer	Total
Seriously limited ability							
Number	2	0	0	2	11	0	15
Percent	13.3	0	0	13.3	73.4	0	100
Moderately limited ability							
Number	9	8	6	26	4	0	53
Percent	17.0	15.1	11.3	49.1	7.5	0	100
Slightly limited ability							
Number	54	12	14	22	6	0	108
Percent	50.0	11.0	13.0	20.4	5.6	0	100
No incapacity							
Number	97	8	9	12	0	1	127
Percent	76.4	6.3	7.1	9.4	0	0.8	100
Total							
Number	162	28	29	62	21	1	303
Percent	53.5	9.2	9.6	20.5	6.9	0.3	100

*19 persons said they drive to services.

Source: Canadian user survey.

While differences in participation were not great, in most outer area developments less than a third (or a few cases less than 40 percent) of the surveyed residents participated in community organizations even once a month; there were only a few exceptions to this. In comparison, at least half, and often many more, of the surveyed elderly at these downtown developments participated in community organizations at least once a month. However, degree of church attendance and participation in senior citizen centers were about the same for development residents at the two different type locations.

The complaint about inaccessibility was less frequent in the few outer area developments that provided transportation for their residents. One development had its own bus, another used a bus to the subway stop, and a third had access to a bus service of a nearby nursing home; in these particular outer area developments most residents said there was easy access to services, though in reality they did not get out daily to a high degree (less than a third of the residents got out one hour or more daily in two of these developments). Another outer area suburban development proved satisfactory on accessibility for the reason that it was adjacent to a shopping center. Few at this development complained of inaccessibility and two-thirds of the surveyed residents got out daily. Thompson has strongly suggested shopping center areas as locations for elderly housing; she would like shopping center developers to include a site for such housing in their plans.

Another indicator of concern with accessibility among many outer area residents was shown by the fact that some spontaneously mentioned it as an answer to an open-ended question on overall satisfaction with the development; 35 elderly persons gave "conveniently located for getting to important places" as a reason for overall satisfaction; a reason for dissatisfaction that 12 elderly gave was "prefer another location."

When asked to specify about satisfaction with location, the main open-ended answers given on reasons for satisfaction were "close to everything" or "close to shopping," followed by "close to transportation." Other reasons included "close to friends and relatives," or "familiar area," but only a very few gave these. One reason given for dissatisfaction was "too far to store." The comment "close to friends and relatives" should not, however, indicate that access to relatives was a priority to these surveyed elderly, for it was not, as only a few gave it as a reason for satisfaction and even fewer (one) gave it as a reason for dissatisfaction with the development. When asked if they felt it was important to have the development located in the same neighborhood or city that their children live, only 40 percent of those with children said it was very important and 36 percent said somewhat important. Single old people were not any more eager than couples to have their children near; those in poor health, however, were more interested.

Nor do elderly necessarily want all services accessible to them, even though they consider accessibility of services in general important to them. The need may be filled by having a grocery store and medical clinic or offices near. These two facilities/services are the ones that we found surveyed elderly in our Canadian study want most accessible. A similar finding came from the survey of U.S. elderly in private housing participating in the HUD-sponsored housing allowance experiment in eight cities. When asked what special feature they looked for and needed in locating any place to live, well over half of these elderly in the HUD-sponsored experiment said a place convenient to shopping; a smaller group said a place close to a doctor, clinic, hospital; far fewer said accessibility to church or closeness to relatives and friends. The Canadian surveyed elderly were also much less concerned about having the library, senior citizens center, church, or even relatives nearby. In fact, unfortunately, most elderly in the development do not visit these facilities; less than a third used a senior citizen center weekly and only 43 percent attended church weekly. Lawton,[34] likewise, found, in his study of elderly at 12 urban housing sites, that the frequency of use of neighborhood services was low; these elderly went to shops on the average of two times a week.

This does not mean accessibility to these services is not important to satisfy the few that do use them, but it does show the surprisingly low use. Degree of use, of course, also relates to health status, with congregate having residents less likely to use community services. It may also differ by whether the group is one that traditionally has low use or high use of such services. An urbane middle-class group that has always used a library and community social clubs may be expected to have a higher use than a rural elderly group or working-class group that has traditionally made lower use of services and traditionally had the services less accessible. In such cases as the latter, a job of the development, when facilities are nearby, is to encourage use.

One might want to site the development near important services both to encourage use and to avoid providing the services in the development, thus saving in costs. Siting the development near the medical clinic or hospital is considered advantageous, and is recommended by many experts. The one caution in doing this is to put enough of a barrier between the two to avoid identification with the sick atmosphere of the hospital.

Siting the development near a shopping facility again has advantages. Likewise, siting it near a church or senior citizen center is good, for then the recreational activities can be arranged by these groups; in a number of such cases the development is affiliated with the religious group concerned. There are also some disadvantages to depending on these nearby community facilities, as was pointed out above in the section on alternative means of providing facilities.

If the site is an outer area location, one must compensate for this location by having some sort of shop or a grocery delivery service, and by having a medical clinic open once a week or more. One may also need to bring in recreational staff and set up weekly religious services as well as provide beauty-barber shop services and dry cleaning services from outside sources. Since only a few residents may use each of these services, efforts to provide them, while necessary, may be frustrating; some development managers unfortunately just give up on doing it. Ideally, one may want to consider selecting for an outer area development lacking facilities and services the types of tenants who need or use few services or are not strongly inclined to participating in outside organizations. However, this may mean selecting mainly the passive type of elderly or those too incompetent even for activities in the development, and then one gets a dull institutional atmosphere.

Attractive Locations Versus Accessibility

Accessibility to services and facilities is only one dimension of the site location problem. Data from our user survey showed other features of the site must be considered. Some of our downtown residents were dissatisfied with location and at the same time satisfied with accessibility to services. On the other hand, some outer area residents who were dissatisfied with accessibility to services were satisfied with location because there were pleasant surroundings or a pleasing building. In fact, "nice surroundings" was the main reason for satisfaction with the development and this was mainly mentioned by outer area residents; "close to everything" was the second major reason and in this case more downtown residents mentioned it. For example, in one outer area development many were bothered by lack of services, especially lack of an accessible medical office, yet most gave the development a high rating on satisfaction with location. "Pleasant gardens," "nice looking" were some of the comments made about these outer area developments.

Over three-fourths of all downtown interviewed residents were very or somewhat satisfied with location; about a third were "very" satisfied. Yet a slightly higher proportion of residents of outer area or rural developments were very or somewhat satisfied with location; a greater proportion (over half) were "very" satisfied.

Some downtown residents were unhappy about location, even though they had been satisfied with accessibility, because it was a commercial area, there was noise and traffic, or there was a "hustle-bustle" atmosphere; some said it was a bad area. The exact location in a downtown area can influence the response, for some areas suffer much more from these problems than others. This can be illustrated by the fact that while a high proportion of residents in three-fourths of our surveyed downtown developments were satisfied with location, in several downtown developments few were satisfied. For one, the major reason these surveyed residents were not satisfied was that the residents would "like nicer surroundings"; at another, it was this reason plus the fact "they want a location free of noise" or "they were afraid to go out at night." At a third downtown development, many again mentioned noise. In the outer area developments, where many were dissatisfied with location, the main reason was "far from stores" in all cases. At the same time the main reason residents in downtown developments were satisfied, especially in the developments where there was a high degree of satisfaction, was that they were close to everything or to some particular service.

Another reason for satisfaction with location, or dissatisfaction, can relate to whether the residents of a neighborhood are mainly of one's own age group. While this was not mentioned in open-ended questions, when specifically asked, 43 percent of these interviewed elderly said they preferred to live in an area where there was not an age mix; 18 percent said they would somewhat prefer an age mix and only 7 percent said they would definitely prefer an age mix; 23 percent said they did not care and 9 percent gave no answer (see Table 8.5). This would indicate these elderly would prefer an inner area with a concentration of elderly rather than a suburban area with many children.

In fact, from the manager survey we find over a third of these downtown developments were characterized by their managers as areas with a concentration of elderly, while a much smaller proportion of the suburban, rural, or even older residential area developments were characterized by their managers as being neighborhoods of mostly elderly; rather, they were predominantly areas of "mostly families with children," with less than a fifth of the managers in any of these areas saying they were neighborhoods of "mostly elderly." A last interesting finding from our survey in this regard was that satisfaction with location did not always conform with overall satisfaction with the development, indicating again that other features of the development can make up for location, such as a good building, pleasant staff, and the already mentioned access to services and existence of these services in the development. For example, many residents who expressed considerable dissatisfaction with the location of one downtown development gave the same development an above-average rating for general satisfaction; on the contrary, resi-

TABLE 8.5

Preference Concerning Residence in Same Building or Same Area
with Families and People of Different Ages

Preference	In Same Building	In Same Area
Definitely prefer age mix		
Number	7	20
Percent	2.3	6.6
Somewhat prefer age mix		
Number	25	55
Percent	8.3	18.2
Somewhat prefer own age		
Number	213	71
Percent	70.3	23.4
Definitely prefer own age		
Number	58	131
Percent	19.1	43.2
No answer		
Number	—	26
Percent	—	8.6
Total		
Number	303	303
Percent	100	100

Source: Canadian user survey.

dents of another downtown development in the same city did just the
opposite—they approved of the location but were generally dissatisfied
with the development.

Location: A Multidimensional Problem

Our findings from the Canadian study indicate there are many
dimensions to the location problem. Some further general comments
may provide an expanded view of the complexities.

Inner city areas give the elderly the advantage of accessibility,
good transportation, familiarity, with possibly friends and relatives
nearby; however, as the above data point out, there can be problems
of being in areas of too much traffic and noise and, above all, of being in deteriorated slum locations. In the United States especially,
an inner city area can mean an area where bars predominate, where

teenage youth loiter, and where the crime rate is so high that the security of the elderly is very much threatened. Several robberies or muggings can make the elderly decide not to go outside the development even in the daytime. There can also be the fear of intruders in the development. As noted previously, at one West Coast inner city elderly public housing development, in an area of transients and skid row types, the situation of intruders got so bad, with muggings and even murder occurring, that residents demanded security guards and a variety of security measures. The answer obviously is not to build in such an area, even if the land is cheaper or more available. Sometimes urban renewal areas, or any type of area where demolition is under way, offer not only the unpleasant view of half-vacated buildings and vacant lots and possibly the noise of demolition but also the lack of safety of a barren area with few pedestrians. The author has seen an elderly development in such a location; it had the looks of a fortress surrounded by a depressing wasteland.

In some cases public housing authorities have found themselves stuck with just such sites. Historically, as the author described in "Stigma and Public Housing,"[35] local communities have resisted the location of public housing on land that was considered to any degree desirable. Public housing was put next to industrial plants, with their insidious smell, in ravines, in isolated spots and, of course, generally in slum areas. While public housing for the elderly has fared somewhat better, there still has been considerable resistance by middle-class residents to putting public housing for the elderly or even elderly nonprofit developments in their area. The stigma of public housing is still strong. In fact, in the 1974 HUD-sponsored housing allowance study, many elderly surveyed in private units said they did not want to live in public housing, even though this particular group was willing to apply for a housing allowance subsidy.

While the resistance to elderly public housing has been lower in many small towns than in cities, possibly because they know the potential residents or are not as zoning conscious, it has been a problem in the suburbs. Zoning ordinances have also often made it more difficult for congregate housing to locate in residential areas.

Public housing authorities have sometimes placed elderly housing adjacent to family public housing. This has a number of problems that indicate it is not advisable. As reported in our case study on Culloden Court, Vancouver, the many children in the family units can harass the elderly in a variety of ways and may try to dominate the project's few facilities, in this case the community room. A worse situation is where the elderly have one floor in a public housing building otherwise occupied by families, as in the case of one White Plains, New York, housing project. There the teenage children monopolize the elevator and the lobby and occasionally harass elderly in both places.

The elderly themselves, as mentioned above, would rather not have an age mix in the neighborhood where they live. These Canadian interviewed elderly were also very strongly against sharing their building with persons of other ages and children; 89 percent said they would prefer to live in a building with their own age group (19 percent definitely preferred and 70 percent somewhat preferred their own age group). This does not mean elderly are not interested in watching children if they can do it from a safe distance such as a balcony facing down on a schoolyard or a nursery school, as is occasionally designed.[36] However, in general, having a noisy public school or family public housing next door, with teenagers loitering about the area, is not suitable.

While elderly public housing built in the early 1970s, before the 1973 moratorium slowed down building, was more likely to be scattered and was less likely to be adjacent to family public housing or in the worst inner city areas, there were high-rise projects that were converted from family to elderly public housing and they were often still in undesirable sites.

In addition, many projects were in racially segregated areas. There are dilemmas of placing elderly housing in minority areas. The project has less chance of becoming integrated. White elderly may not want to apply if it is a minority area. And their relatives may discourage them, both because of the area and because of their inaccurate assessment that there will be conflict between black and white residents. No research has shown problems between black and white elderly tenants and studies have in fact shown many friendships across ethnic and racial lines.[37]

Because projects in minority areas have less chance of becoming integrated, HUD has been reluctant to approve use of such sites. Yet it has been hard to get other sites, and the need for this housing for minority elderly is especially great. Also, nonprofit groups sponsoring Section 202 and, in the past, Section 236 housing are sometimes minority churches and should have the right to build in their own neighborhoods.

Inner city areas in transition from white to minority areas can also be a problem as this change can cause tension for elderly residents. If these elderly formerly lived in the area they have nostalgia for the neighborhood as it was and are bothered by the changes taking place. If families with many children move into the houses around them, tensions can develop, as Sterne, Phillips, and Rabushka point out for a Rochester inner city area in The Urban Elderly Poor.[38]

If there is a high crime rate in a minority area, as there is in most inner city areas, whether white or minority, then tensions are further increased.

Use of alternative of siting elderly subsidized housing in white nonslum areas has increased. In fact, elderly integrated housing has had better luck than family conventional housing in getting in white areas or in integrated areas, just as leased public housing in some places, such as San Francisco, has been well represented in white areas, even though a number of tenants are black, as Peel, Pickett, and Buehl point out in the Stanford Law Review.[39]

A main consideration one should have in looking for a site is whether the neighborhood is a respectable one, one that the elderly can feel proud of or not ashamed to tell their relatives and friends they are in. When given a chance, elderly in slum areas, if at all inclined to move, are likely to move out of such areas to better neighborhoods; for example, of elderly on the experimental housing allowance who did move, most moved to better neighborhoods. At the same time studies show elderly do not want to move long distances to unknown areas. Urban housing groups in the United States and Britain that have built elderly housing for their applicants in resorts a long way from their city have gotten mixed results.* Some elderly do not want to move that far away.

Many elderly prefer to stay close to the area where they always lived. The housing authority or nonprofit group thus has the difficult job of locating a site in a safe respectable neighborhood that still is accessible to services and transportation and close to landmarks familiar to these elderly. In most cities such areas exist, but land in such respectable inner area locations is not cheap. The extra land cost and the fight to overcome zoning problems and resident opposition may be, however, worthwhile if this means the elderly get some site features to which they give priority.

These developments can also be landscaped. While outer sites are specifically associated with a parklife atmosphere, green lawns, and in general pleasant surroundings, there is no reason why some lawn and landscaping cannot be done on inner area sites; it certainly is in a number we know of. It may be only a small strip or shrubs inserted in a cement wall but it can give a sense of pride and enjoyment. It may be a small area provided with benches so that the elderly on sunny days can watch passersby.

The development may also be placed adjacent to a small city park, as found in some cases in Europe as well as the United States. A small park area in a nonslum inner city area may be kept secure, both because of size and the many pedestrians passing by and because efforts have been made by the police and the development to keep it

---

*The Greater London Council has had trouble attracting elderly to resort area council housing in some cases; yet the manger of the Brighton Housing Authority, operating in one of the most famous resort areas, told the author in 1967 that there was a high demand for their units.

safe; in other words, it is an activity area under surveillance. It
should hopefully not be an area of dense shrubs or a hangout of teenage gangs.

Studies have found that in general the elderly prefer sites where
there is activity, such as pedestrian traffic, over a quiet pastoral
scene, as Thompson points out.[40] They want to be able to watch the
action even if they can no longer take part in it. Action can be stimu-
lating, as with a park with deer and ducks we found near one Dutch
development.

The site should not be on a slope or a hill where the elderly must
walk up steps or climb a hill when returning from the bus stop. It
should not be at a traffic intersection where one must cross a very
busy street to get to the bus stop or to services, and where chances
of traffic accidents are high.

While all these recommendations on site location are useful,
in the end the development must be located on a site that is financially
within the sponsor's means. Of course in doing this, the sponsor
should calculate the extra costs of having to provide services and
facilities on an isolated site or the cost of having a dissatisfied clientele and possibly a development with a number of units vacant. This
happened to the Minneapolis area congregate development we observed
(Berkshire Home); located in a small town 20 miles from Minneapolis
and located five to ten blocks from a small shopping area, for the
first year it filled only about half of its units. Nor should a slum area
site be accepted because of cheap land (nor urban renewal land in an
undesirable residential or industrial area). However, even with
these setoffs, land cost must be kept in mind as well as zoning regulations (of course, if the land is donated by an individual or organization, this is harder to get around).

One way sponsors find whereby they can justify the more expensive inner area sites is to build high-rise buildings, even though
some would argue that the landscaping around high rise plus the cost
of building high rises push the total cost up. The ideal may be to build
high-density low rise, but this does not always seem architecturally
possible. While high-rise buildings are not considered the most desirable type, both the sponsor and the elderly themselves may see it
as a tradeoff for being able to locate in an inner city accessible area.

USE OF HIGH-RISE BUILDINGS

The use of high-rise structures for housing developments for
the elderly has been a controversial issue. Popular attention, often
emotionally charged, has been drawn to negative aspects of the quality
of urban life in high rise. The social impact of vertical living environ-

ments has been described in terms of alienation, mental tension and distress, and the destruction of positive family living and child-rearing patterns.[41] High-rise structures have been correlated with density and crowding and these in turn correlated with stress and tension and social pathologies.

The findings quoted in articles condemning high rise have usually been of studies of, first, families living in high rise, and second, mainly poor families living in public housing, as Robert E. Mitchell points out. As he quite rightly reports:

> Often equally high density for the wealthy—such as on
> Miami Beach, Waikiki, or Park Avenue—as well as cam-
> pus dormitories, do not exhibit the same kinds of se-
> verely disturbed social and personal conditions that have
> become associated in the public mind with high rise, high
> density public housing for poor people. To blame these
> social problems on the physical features of housing,
> therefore, is to overlook the problem of poverty, discrimi-
> nation, and family functioning.[42]

In a major Toronto study of middle-class, mainly childless, couples in high rise, with the wife usually employed, findings again do not support the stereotype. William Michelson found that these couples are "no more isolated, according to the various measures, than are those living in other types of dwellings."[43] The high rise may be suitable and satisfactory for those cosmopolitans who want a central location, although not acceptable for families, as Fritz Nigg of Zurich[44] points out.

Gerda R. Wekerle,[45] studying a Chicago high-rise building mainly occupied by singles, found a high degree of interaction among tenants. Here, upper-middle-class, well-educated, single young adults were attracted to this high rise because it had the homogeneous population and the promise of a swinging life style that they wanted.

From these examples, one should agree with Claude S. Fischer, Mark Baldassare, and Richard J. Ofshe[46] that the effects of density are highly dependent on individual, situational (social and architec-tural), and cultural factors. One must, furthermore, concur with Mitchell's conclusion that "there is no evidence that high densities—either on the land or within individual dwelling units—have seriously adverse effects on the emotional or family health of at least several populations that have been studied."[47]

The elderly may be one of these populations. As Wekerle points out, "there are increasingly large numbers of non-family households, both young and old, who reside in high rise apartments, and our knowledge about the suitability of high rise apartments for this segment of the population is almost nonexistent."[48]

An age-segregated environment, we know, appeals to many elderly, as our Canadian research and other studies show; over three-fourths of our surveyed elderly wanted to live in an age-segregated building. Age-segregated high-rise developments may therefore be accepted by many elderly, as our own research and that of Lawton[49] show. In our user survey we asked respondents to give their reaction to positive and negative attitudinal statements about high rise. Analysis was done in terms of comparing the responses of the 176 living in high-rise buildings (here defined as over five floors high) and the 127 living in low-rise buildings. Two-thirds in high rise had a totally or somewhat positive attitude to high rise; only 16 percent of those in low rise did.

The disadvantages of living in high rise were mentioned by a few, with almost a fifth of the total sample expressing the commonly heard disadvantage: "Many old people fear heights" and thus do not care to live high above the ground; and almost a fifth of the group said a disadvantage was that "poor elevator services in high rise force residents to climb stairs." And this is supported by Lawton,[50] who says, from his interviews, that some old people are genuinely phobic about living above the ground level and have a strong aversion to high-rise living, and some cannot bring themselves to ride an elevator. He adds that in percentage terms, their number is small, and we also found this.

Besides this psychological concern about heights and possibly density, another psychological disadvantage noted by a few was that "high rise produces a claustrophobic feeling"; commonly mentioned are "the danger of fires and difficulties for firemen," or the fact that in high rise "access to outdoors is difficult." This problem certainly exists, but a good sprinkler system, use of fireproof materials, and the provision of several elevators can lessen it.

Another often-heard complaint, that in high rise it is hard to control the access to the building and therefore there is more of a security problem,[51] was not mentioned by our Canadian elderly. Newman,[52] in his negative report on crime in high rise, brings this up but then relates it to families with many children living in high rise and to certain features of modern architectural design, such as long corridors and outside areas that cannot be surveyed by residents. Lawton says "if we assume that a project will serve only the elderly, so far as we know there is no clear evidence to favor one or the other type of structure for security purposes. If a single individual, such as a security guard, is assigned the job of monitoring access to the project, he will probably be more effective in a high rise than patrolling the wider expanses of a low rise project."[53] One can also add that there are less chances of peeping toms in high rise as compared to low-rise buildings, as was found in a British high-rise study.[54]

More respondents in our sample gave a positive than negative reaction to high rise. The main advantages they saw, above all, with a fourth of the group mentioning each, were that "the building does have maintenance services done for you" and "the building takes less land, so is closer into the city." Other advantages related to these, mentioned by a few, were that high rise was "closer to relatives" and "cheaper." Some of the elderly saw this tradeoff of living in high rise in order to be in a central location where land is expensive and scarce and thus where building vertically may be necessary.

The fact that the elderly living in high rise were more likely. feel they were accessible to services than those living in low-rise housing may be a verification that high rise allowed them a central location. Almost two-thirds in high rise, but only slightly over a third in low rise, said all services were easily accessible.

High-rise tenants were also somewhat more likely to say they were satisfied with location, when specifically asked about this, than was true for low-rise tenants, who were often living in suburban, fringe, or rural areas. Well over half of the high-rise residents were very satisfied with location.

Another advantage our users saw in high rise was that it "provides more company" as well as being closer to friends and relatives. These comments were probably due to the size of the development and its location. Analysis of social participation data showed, first, those living in high-rise buildings were slightly more active in outside community organizations than those living in low rise. Second, somewhat fewer of those in high rise said they never went out, though both groups were as likely to get out one hour or more daily. This contradicts Lawton's finding that "other things being equal, tenants in low rise buildings seem to be more likely to leave the premises and engage in more outwardly-directed activity."[55]

Our data also showed that in reality those in high rise did not participate more in the development than those in low rise, even though a fair degree of contact among high-rise elderly tenants did take place. When asked, first, if they had made many, some, or hardly any friends in the development, only a third of the high-rise tenants said "many friends" while half of the low-rise development residents did. Second, low-rise residents were slightly more likely to visit friends in the development daily or even weekly. This could be because more low-rise residents were in rural developments, where neighbors are usually considered more friendly.

Interestingly, Lawton feels "there seems to be greater participation in on-site activity programs in high rise buildings."[56] Regardless of whether participation is slightly higher in high rise or low rise, the fact is that few of these residents are socially isolated and therefore do not fit the stereotype of high-rise tenants.

Other advantages of high rise mentioned were "more services given" and, related to this, the already covered comment, made by a fourth, that maintenance service is done for them. This is more likely related to the size of the building than to the vertical structure. A large building is more likely to have services and staff. When specifically asked about size, respondents who lived in medium-size high rise were slightly more likely to say the size was "all right" rather than the building was "too large" or "small," as compared to those in low rise, who were often in small buildings that some felt were too small, mainly because there were few services or not enough people to interact with. Since many of the high-rise developments were congregate, they had many staff and services.

Other advantages of high rise mentioned were that residents had a "good view" and "fresh air." Many elderly enjoy the city view. At the same time a very few were bothered that they could not walk out on a lawn or have a garden. However, it need not be assumed all elderly want to garden. In fact, 27 percent of all respondents said a garden plot was available but only 10 percent used them. Poor health was a main reason for not using them.

Another advantage of high rise was it allowed privacy, was quiet, and had less noise than low rise. On a question on satisfaction with privacy, a considerably higher proportion in high rise than in low rise felt privacy was very satisfactory. In a British study[57] of families living in high rise, the respondents again gave privacy as one advantage of living in high rise; they did not like the peeping toms they sometimes got when occupying a ground floor apartment.

These various advantages were much more likely to be given by those elderly now living in high rise than those in low rise, for, as already mentioned, two-thirds of those living in high rise had a totally or somewhat positive attitude toward high rise, as indicated in response to four attitude statements, while only 16 percent in low rise did. The interviewers felt that those living in low-rise housing, often in small towns, had little knowledge of or experience with high-rise living; many had probably never been in such a building. This also accounts for the large "don't know" group on these statements (about a fifth of the total group). This difference of opinion was also registered for the two positive statements individually—the statements being that "high-rise buildings have many advantages for senior citizens" and "high-rise buildings are ideal places for senior citizens to live"; on both, half of those in high rise agreed, but less than one-fifth in low rise did (see Table 8.6).

On the two negative statements, less than a fourth of high-rise residents agreed; these were that "most senior citizens prefer not to live in high-rise buildings" and "high-rise buildings are an unsatisfactory place for senior citizens to live in." Almost two-thirds of the elderly in low-rise buildings did agree with these statements.

TABLE 8.6

Overall Negative or Positive Opinion about High-Rise Buildings,
by Size of Development

| | Size of Development | | | |
Opinion	Large	Medium	Small	All
Totally negative				
Number	20	17	17	54
Percent	14.6	19.2	22.0	17.8
Somewhat negative				
Number	18	13	20	51
Percent	13.1	14.6	26.0	16.8
Mixed feelings				
Number	12	11	14	37
Percent	8.8	12.4	18.2	12.2
Somewhat favorable				
Number	35	22	6	63
Percent	25.5	24.8	7.8	20.8
Very favorable				
Number	48	19	9	76
Percent	35.0	21.3	11.7	25.1
No answer				
Number	4	7	11	22
Percent	2.9	7.7	14.3	7.3
Total				
Number	137	89	77	303
Percent	100	100	100	100

Source: Canadian user survey.

These findings are not surprising. Lawton found the same.
He says that "people with earlier high rise living experience strongly
prefer to live in high rise projects for the elderly" and that "the very
great majority of people who move into a high rise building end up
strongly liking this arrangement"; but he also says that "similarly,
the great majority who move into low rise projects prefer that kind
of living"; he then reports that "a significant minority of people have
some question as to whether they will be comfortable in high rise
buildings" and that "another larger minority [or even perhaps a majority?] of people would not actively choose high rise living if they
had completely free choice."[58]

But when they actually live in high rise, many seem satisfied. A Glasgow, Scotland, research team[59] did a study of tenants in high flats; they found among the elderly in their group, 94 percent were satisfied with their home, though one problem for some was loneliness.

Of our users, those in high rise were more likely to be in general satisfied with the development than were those in low rise; there was a 12 percent difference between the two groups.

In sum, one can say there are mixed feelings about high rise, but many elderly are willing to live in such and see a number of advantages.

NOTES

1. U.S. Department of Housing and Urban Development, HUD Handbook: Community Service Functions in the Area Insuring Office (Washington, D.C.: Government Printing Office, December 1974).

2. U.S. Department of Housing and Urban Development, Management of Congregate Housing: HUD Guidelines (Washington, D.C.: Government Printing Office, 1972), pp. 4, 14.

3. Marie McGuire Thompson, Design of Housing for the Elderly (Washington, D.C.: National Association of Housing and Urban Redevelopment Officials, 1972), pp. 15-17; M. Powell Lawton, Planning and Managing Housing for the Elderly (New York: John Wiley and Sons, 1975), pp. 106-11, 295-97.

4. Interview with James Frush, president, Retirement Residences, July 24, 1976.

5. Testimony by Frederic Fay, director, Richmond (Virginia) Redevelopment and Housing Authority, in Adequacy of Federal Response to Housing Needs of Older Americans, Hearings, U.S. Congress, Senate, Special Committee on Aging, 94th Cong., 1st sess., October 1975, pt. 14, p. 1003.

6. Testimony by Marie McGuire Thompson, in Adequacy of Federal Response to Housing Needs of Older Americans, pt. 13, p. 902.

7. Ibid.

8. Testimony by Matthew Tayback, in Adequacy of Federal Response to Housing Needs of Older Americans, pt. 13, p. 933.

9. Testimony by Kallia Bokser, in Adequacy of Federal Response to Housing Needs of Older Americans, pt. 13, p. 916.

10. Thompson, in Adequacy of Federal Response to Housing Needs of Older Americans, pt. 13, p. 904.

11. Silverman, in Adequacy of Federal Response to Housing Needs of Older Americans, pt. 14, p. 995.

12. Lawton, Planning and Managing Housing for the Elderly, pp. 106-07.

13. Ernest Noam, Homes for the Aged: Supervision and Standards: A Report on the Legal Situation in European Countries (Washington, D.C.: U.S. Department of Health, Education and Welfare, Administration on Aging, 1975), p. 6.

14. Ibid.

15. Elizabeth Huttman, "Social Policy for Housing the Elderly" (paper presented at Society for Study of Social Problems meetings, San Francisco, August 1975), p. 5.

16. Interview with Frush, July 24, 1976.

17. Noam, Homes for the Aged, p. 4.

18. Ibid., p. 5.

19. Testimony by Robert McCann, director, Manchester (New Hampshire) Housing Authority, in Adequacy of Federal Response to Housing Needs of Older Americans, pt. 13, p. 923.

20. Lawton, Planning and Managing Housing for the Elderly.

21. Ibid., p. 264.

22. Ibid., p. 306.

23. Ibid.

24. Ibid.

25. Frances M. Carp, "Congregate Housing: Concept and Role" (paper presented at National Conference on Congregate Housing for Older People, Washington, D.C., November 11-12, 1975), p. 15.

26. Testimony by Wilma Donahue, Adequacy of Federal Response to Housing Needs of Older Americans, pt. 13, p. 895.

27. Ibid.

28. Marie McGuire Thompson, "Management of Congregate Housing" (paper presented at National Conference on Congregate Housing for Older People, Washington, D.C., November 11-12, 1975), pp. 1-2.

29. Carp, "Congregate Housing," p. 14.

30. Marie McGuire Thompson, "Congregate Housing for Older Adults: A Working Paper" (presented to U.S. Congress, Senate, Special Committee on Aging, 94th Cong., 1st sess., 1975), pp. 23-24.

31. J. P. Huttman and E. D. Huttman, "Size, Height and Location as Land Use Issues in Provision of Housing for Ambulatory Elderly," in Papers and Proceedings of Third Pacific Regional Science Meetings (August 1973) (Toyko, 1976).

32. Lawton, Planning and Managing Housing for the Elderly, p. 191.

33. Noam, Homes for the Aged, p. 6.

34. Lawton, Planning and Managing Housing for Elderly, p. 88.

35. Elizabeth Huttman, "Stigma and Public Housing" (Ph.D. diss. University of California, Berkeley, 1969), chap. 6.

36. Lawton, Planning and Managing Housing for Elderly, p. 97.

37. Ibid., p. 93.

38. Richard Sterne, James Phillips, and Alvin Rabushka, The Urban Elderly Poor (Lexington, Mass.: Lexington Books, 1974), p. 23.

39. Norman Peel, Garth Pickett, and Stephen Buehl, "Racial Discrimination in Public Housing Site Selection," Stanford Law Review 23 (November 1970): 66-147.

40. Thompson, Design of Housing for the Elderly, pp. 5-6.

41. Daniel Cappon, "Mental Health in the High Rise," Canadian Journal of Public Health 62 (September-October, 1971): 426-31; D. M. Fanning, "Families in Flats," British Medical Journal 4 (November 18, 1967): 382-86; Ann Stevenson, Elaine Martin, and Judith O'Neill, High Living: A Study of Family Life in Flats (Melbourne: Melbourne University Press, 1967).

42. Robert E. Mitchell, "Misconceptions about Man-Made Space: In Partial Defense of High Density Housing," The Family Coordinator 23, no. 1 (January 1974): 52.

43. William Michelson, "The Reconciliation of 'Subjective' and 'Objective' Data on Community Environment: The Case of Social Contact in High Rise Apartments" (paper presented at American Sociological Association meetings, New York, September 1973), p. 24.

44. Fritz Nigg, quoted in Elizabeth Hunn and Ruedi Jost, "Sind Wohntürme das Höchste oder die Höhe?" Schweizer Illustrierte 28 (July 5, 1976): 21-23.

45. Gerda R. Wekerle, "Vertical Village: Social Contacts in a Singles Highrise Complex" (paper presented at the American Sociological Association meetings, San Francisco, August 1975).

46. Claude S. Fischer, Mark Baldassare, and Richard J. Ofshe, "Crowding Studies and Urban Life: A Critical Review," in American Institute of Planners Journal 41, no. 6 (November 1975): 406-17.

47. Mitchell, "Misconceptions about Man-Made Space," p. 55.

48. Wekerle, "Vertical Village," p. 2.

49. Lawton, Planning and Managing Housing for the Elderly, p. 142.

50. Ibid.

51. Ibid.

52. Oscar Newman, Defensible Space: Crime Prevention Through Urban Design (New York: Macmillan, 1972).

53. Lawton, Planning and Managing Housing for the Elderly, p. 141.

54. Joan Ash and Michael Burbridge, Families at High Density: A Study of Estates in Leeds, Liverpool and London (London: Her Majesty's Stationery Office, Ministry of Housing and Local Government, 1970).

55. Lawton, Planning and Managing Housing for the Elderly, p. 142.

56. Ibid.

57. Ash and Burbridge, Families at High Density, p. 29.

58. Ibid.

59. Pearl Jephcott, with Hilary Robinson, Homes in High Flats, University of Glasgow Social and Economic Studies, Occasional Papers, no. 13 (Edinburgh: Oliver and Boyd, 1971).

9

SATELLITE CENTRAL, OAKLAND, CALIFORNIA

Satellite Central, a Section 236 project with rent supplement program, is one of 11 nonprofit elderly complexes run by Satellite Senior Homes, a church-oriented organization operating in Oakland and adjacent communities. This development, built in 1970, has 151 units, of which 75 are efficiency, 42 are jumbo studios, and 34 one-bedroom apartments; it has 160 residents. Satellite Central serves two meals on weekdays and provides a variety of services.

Satellite Central is a ten-story high-rise building in downtown Oakland, on a side street only one to two blocks away from the main shopping area. It is close to two churches, the YMCA, and a major department store. The Greyhound bus depot is down the block and bus stops for local buses are within a block. Clinics, barber shops, and movie theaters are a short walk away. This extreme accessibility is appreciated by many residents; a number said they came to the development, or they were satisfied with it, because of its location and accessibility to stores and services. Others said they liked it because it was in a familiar area.

Satellite Central has mainly healthy ambulatory elderly. Yet it offers them a semicongregate arrangement. It has a noon meal service, cafeteria style, that offers the residents the option of using or not using the service as well as the option of buying whatever they want; outsiders may also come in to use this cafeteria at noon, as a number of community elderly do. The Satellite Central also serves an evening meal for its own tenants; the price of this waitress-service meal is included in the tenants' rent. Salt-free diets are prepared. As for breakfast, the residents must use their kitchenettes.

Both the noon and evening meals are only available Monday through Friday. Some residents who do not have relatives in the area occasionally cook together on weekends. Since development residents are mainly single and a number are widowers, they are the type of elderly who appreciate having meals prepared for them. These residents have a small kitchenette in the efficiency or jumbo studio, or a full kitchen in the one-bedroom apartment.

Other facilities Satellite Central has include a laundry room on the tenth floor, a library adjacent to the lobby, and a large activities room on that floor, which is used for classes, playing cards, movies, special events, and visiting. In the basement there is also a recreation room used for art classes and for special clinics. The lobby is large enough to also act as a small lounge, and a number of elderly sit here before or after meals. Adjacent to it is a mailbox-bulletin board area where coming events in the building and in the community are announced. This board acts as an information and referral source; there is also a list of telephone numbers that the tenants can call for referral.

The development also has an outside roof garden with a magnificent view of the Bay Area, a tenth-floor sitting area, and a balcony along one side of the second floor. Some individual apartments also have their own balcony. There are also parking spaces for the residents who have cars. There is a patio area outside the dining room, and that has a shuffleboard court.

Satellite Central has a variety of activities going on in its facilities. It serves as the meeting place or center for a number of community activities; for example, the Senior Non-Partisan Legislative Group runs its monthly meetings there, with a number of residents taking part. Tours for Oakland seniors, run by the city Recreation Department, also operate out of the development, with an office located there. The recreation coordinator for the development, paid by the Recreation Department and school district, spends considerable time there, although she also has other assignments.

A wide variety of classes and programs are held in the development. On almost every weekday afternoon and some evenings there are classes, such as ceramics, weaving, painting, crochet, creative writing, English, lip reading, history, religion of the world, dressmaking. The instructors come from different educational and recreational resources in the area, such as the local junior college adult education program. There are bingos weekly, bridge games, and such.

Special events include a monthly birthday dinner party with decorations prepared by the dining room staff, holiday parties, and movies. The development's Tenant Association holds a monthly meeting, at which time there is a special event arranged by residents

of a particular floor of the development; each month a different floor
is responsible. In this way residents have a chance for leadership
and participation in arranging their own recreation.

In addition to this, tenants take part in the tours and other activities run by the many active senior citizen organizations and agencies in the city. The development's central location means easy access to these, as well as to religious services.

Special transportation services are also available from the
community, even though public transportation is good and location
makes access to services excellent. A specially run shopping service of the Catholic church takes the residents to a large supermarket
every two weeks.

Social and legal counseling is done by a social worker from a
local agency dealing with the elderly; this person comes by appointment and deals with such problems as lost checks. Her visits are
fairly frequent. A homemaker service is also available from a community agency.

Certain medical services are also available in the development.
A podiatrist comes in once every two weeks. A public health nurse
runs a blood pressure clinic once a month, and there is a screening-
of-the-eyes clinic once a month. Several residents have individual
visits from nurses. In addition, there are a number of medical facilities nearby. There is no nurse or doctor on staff.

While the residents are generally in good health, a few have
been found sick in their apartment; some are in their eighties and
even nineties. The development security system to meet medical
emergencies takes several forms. Each apartment has an emergency
alarm system that the elderly person can activate in his bedroom or
toilet; staff is available on a 24-hour basis to cover this. An assistant manager, an elderly resident, covers the 5 p.m.-to-8 a.m. period weekdays and gives complete coverage on weekends. This assistant manager also checks people out for weekend or other visits and
generally keeps track of the residents' whereabouts. She is backed
up by a receptionist who also lives in the building.

Each floor also has two resident floor managers whose job is
to keep in contact with tenants on that floor, tell the management
about tenant needs, and organize parties when the floor's turn comes
up. Since most residents are single, these security measures are
especially welcome.

To avoid accidents, safety design features are also built into
each apartment. There are grab rails and exhaust fans in the bathrooms; stove and carpet have been chosen for safety features.

Another type of security system is in terms of keeping out intruders in this inner city area. The doors of the development are
locked at 5 p.m. After that, any visitor must work through the inter-

com system at the entrance, identifying himself to the resident. Security is also assisted by the fact that the lobby is a heavily used sitting area; residents sitting there can readily identify intruders.

The staff of this 151-unit development is small, considering all the services offered. There is the manager, the manager's secretary, the assistant manager (who is an elderly resident), a receptionist (again a resident), dining room-kitchen staff, and a maintenance staff. The recreational, educational, and medical visitation staff are all provided by other sources. Some tasks are done by the over-all organization for the 11 Satellite senior homes.

These apartments rent for reasonable amounts, even though the rent includes utilities and $45 for the evening meals for a month, as of 1975. This is partly because, as HUD Section 236 subsidized housing, the development's mortgage is at a below market interest rate, but also because the development has been able to get outside funding for many services. The rent of these unfurnished apartments varies not only by whether they are efficiency or jumbo studios, but by floor and by whether they have a balcony. Out of the approximately 160 residents, 30 are on rent supplement, meaning they pay only 25 percent of their income for rent, and the rest of the rent is paid by HUD under this rent supplement program. There is an income limit for residency in any of the units but it is high enough to allow most moderate-income elderly to be eligible (it was $9,500 in August 1976).

SUMMERSET COURT, SUMMERSIDE, PRINCE EDWARD ISLAND, MARITIMES

Summerset Court is a small elderly public housing apartment development in a rural area. It is located a mile from central Summerside, a town of 11,000 on Prince Edward Island, Maritimes. A main feature of the development is that it is adjacent to the Department of Welfare's Manor Special Care Home. It is a quarter mile farther out than the public hospital. Nearby is a small supermarket and a high school; a little farther out is a medical clinic. It is in an area of family homes.

This small development was built in two stages. The first part consists of five motel-type buildings of four apartments each, or a total of 20 units, plus laundry facilities. The other part is across a minor secondary road. It is a single building with 22 apartments and a recreation room and an adjacent laundry room; most of these units are bachelor apartments, while all the units in the first-stage project are one-bedroom apartments. In both parts of the development the apartments have private exterior entrances, but in the stage-two building they also have back doors opening on to a common enclosed hallway.

The residents, at the time of this study, were mainly aged 75 to 79 and their health was quite good, with two-thirds having no incapacity at all. However, some units were vacant while the resident was in the hospital or convalescing with a relative. Half of those interviewed were widows of farmers; because of this, many had relatives ten or more miles away from the development rather than in the town, but they did have a fair degree of contact with them, at least by phone, in many cases. Because of being farmer's wives, most had some income beyond the pension.

The development had no on-site manager or maintenance man at the time of the study. Maintenance was done by the Prince Edward Island Housing Authority's roving crew. Because of this, residents complained it took a long time to have minor repairs attended to. Management of the development was done from the central office of the housing authority, 40 miles away in Charlottetown; the supervisor for the development had many other jobs, with only 15 percent of his work load devoted to all senior citizen buildings on the island. Once a month, one of the supervisor's staff members came out from Charlottetown to collect the rents, and this provided some degree of contact with the residents, although at the time of the study it was found that the normal practice was for the residents to leave their rent for the collector with the manager of the adjacent Manor Special Care Home.

This housing authority, according to the supervisor of housing interviewed at the time, felt its main job was to provide shelter and it could not be involved with seeing that services or facilities were provided. At that time the housing authority was even turning away from the idea of including a recreation room in its elderly projects. The rationale was that there was such a need for decent accommodations on the island that the money should be spent in that way. The housing was usually better than what the person had come from.

The development at the time of the study did have a recreational program running in its recreation room. This new addition was due to the efforts of staff of the island's Rural Development Council to set up senior citizen clubs, with one of their main aims being to help elderly learn how to get information and to solve problems. The Summerset Court club held a weekly sewing circle, informal sing-songs, and monthly business meetings.

Another source for recreational activities was the adjacent Manor, which had a fairly organized program of entertainment. These included weekly singsongs, card nights, bingo games, monthly birthday parties, special holiday parties, and special concerts. Since 43 residents of this special care home were ambulatory, a fair number attended. Tenants of the Summerset apartments were invited to attend, and some did attend, mainly special programs. Half interviewed said they attended some events, sometimes. Some of the residents of the stage-one buildings did not attend for the same reasons they did not attend events in their own project's recreation room; that is, they did not want to go out and cross the street in the night air or even daytime, especially in winter.

The Manor also invited the Summerset apartment residents to use its dining room, charging them only a small amount for meals, and some occasionally did, usually on Sundays. However, most of the interviewed apartment residents indicated they would rather cook for themselves. Some of the Summerset residents also occasionally used the Manor's library.

The administrator of this Department of Welfare special care home probably had more contact with these Summerset apartment residents than any other professional. He saw them when they left their rent with him each month. He counseled them on problems and acted as liaison between them and the project's owner, the housing authority in Charlottetown.

The main contribution the Manor made to the lives of these elderly apartment residents, however, was that it provided a bus to take them the mile to the downtown area. This minibus made seven or so trips a day from 9 a.m. to 5 p.m. on weekdays; at the time of the study, there was no charge to the Summerset apartment residents. Like all the other aspects of the relationship between the Manor and Summerset, at that time this was an informal arrangement. Since the Manor was a Department of Welfare endeavor, there may have been more incentive than if it was nonprofit or a private nursing home. This bus was very much appreciated because there was no public bus service to the project area at that time. However, because this transportation service did not operate nights, or weekends, the residents' activities at these times were curtailed, including church attendance (although some churches picked up their parishioners on Sunday morning). This made some interviewed residents feel isolated. They may have tried to compensate with a heavy visiting pattern in the development; most surveyed tenants said they visited daily within the development, whereas they visited monthly with friends outside the development. This may have been helped by the fact that it was a small development in a rural area, where friendliness is normal. These elderly's isolation may also have been decreased by the fact that they had an emergency alarm system in each apartment, giving some security in case of health emergencies. In such emergencies they of course were also assured of possible assistance from the adjacent special care home, the public hospital a quarter mile away, or even the medical clinic a quarter mile in the other direction.

At the time of the study the lack of a visiting public health nurse to serve these residents on a regular basis in their own homes was,

however, felt to be a shortcoming of the development by several interviewed sources. It was felt some residents who were in the hospital
or convalescing with relatives could possibly have been back in the
development if such a nursing service existed.

When residents' health problems became serious, their alternative was to move into the adjacent Manor Special Care Home. The
Manor tried to give Summerset residents priority in getting in. Interviewed Summerset residents did not mind having a medical care
unit next to them, when specifically asked. All of them were aware
of the levels of care it offered and most named the Manor as the
place they would move to from their apartments.

There is no question that having this special care home adjacent
to the apartment complex and having an administrator and staff who
were willing to welcome to their facilities these apartment users, and
even allow them to use the bus services, made life much more agree-
able in this development. Without such, the fact that these apartment
residents were in a project one mile out of town, not near a public
bus system, not provided with community or development services,
and without staff, might have been intolerable. In this small town
these informal arrangements between the two institutions seemed to
have helped this situation.

FINNISH-CANADIAN REST HOME, VANCOUVER, BRITISH COLUMBIA

The Finnish-Canadian Rest Home is a multilevel nonprofit development in Vancouver, with capital cost assistance by the national
government. It has a congregate wing that houses approximately 55
residents in its mainly single rooms; it has a dining room. The
home's other three buildings contain 93 mainly bachelor apartments,
housing 105 residents. This complex was built in 1963 by the Finnish-
Canadian Rest Home Society, representing 1,100 members of the Finnish community, to meet the needs of their elderly. This development
did not fully cover the need because it lacked a nursing wing, which
by 1972, when we interviewed the management, they considered very
necessary. To remedy this, in 1974 the society built a second development, Finnish Manor, in nearby Burnaby, which includes a 60-bed
nursing unit and 48 apartments as well as a modern auditorium.

This case study is on the first development, but because the two
developments have joint activities and are run by the same society,
mention will also be made of the second.

The Vancouver complex is in a pleasant residential area of
single-family dwelling units about a half-hour bus trip from downtown
Vancouver. On the same street are two other ethnic rest homes. The

complex is pleasantly landscaped and is a well-maintained set of four buildings going down a slope. The three apartment buildings have three floors each; they each have a lobby and a laundry and a basement recreation room used for tenant parties and some storage.

The congregate two-story, two-wing building is the main hub of the development. It is where the complex office is and where rents are paid. It contains a number of well-maintained facilities, houses a number of services, and is the locale of the sizable development staff. It houses the more dependent residents needing congregate care. In contrast, the apartment buildings house mainly well elderly who are quite independent and active and who go their own way; in many cases they have little to do with the congregate building, even though they can take meals there if they so wish and can join in the activities program.

The staff includes a manager and a number of kitchen, house-keeping, and maintenance workers, around ten in all; the nursing unit has 23. The society's board of directors is also active in development operation. This building has a lobby, a lounge off the dining room, a library, a recreation room, a downstairs meeting and recreation room, a sauna, and laundry facilities. The dining room is sometimes used as an auditorium for special events.

At the time of our study (1972-73), the complex was the center of Finnish-Canadian activities in Vancouver, and there were many special events for the whole Finnish community held at the development. A number of outsiders from the Finnish community always attended these special events, which included concerts and such by touring Finnish groups. The members also ran a number of events there. The women ran occasional teas (six or so a year) there for the whole Finnish community. Religious services in Finnish for the whole community were held there on Sundays, usually with coffee or tea following the service. These volunteer women also organized outdoor summer picnics on the pleasant development grounds. To the local Finnish-Canadians, then, it is their center, and they expect to move there when age, health, and general need dictate such. The men of the society helped in the building and especially landscaping and maintaining of the development. The apartment residents have also helped with the maintenance. The society's women made the curtains for this elderly housing.

In 1974 these volunteers began helping on the new complex. Since completed, the community-development activities such as concerts of out-of-town Finnish groups or holiday events have been held in the auditorium of the new complex, and this continues. A free bus service of the society takes the residents of the Vancouver development over to the new Burnaby complex for these and other activities as well as shopping.

It is through this society's efforts that management has not only been able to build and run an attractive initial development, with many apartments and a congregate wing, but has been able to add to their earlier effort, by building a new complex in Burnaby (of 48 more apartment units and a nursing unit of 60 beds). Management is especially proud of this, because when the author visited the home in 1972, a major long-time concern had been to add a nursing unit. They felt many of their present congregate residents would soon need such, as well as Finnish-Canadians in the community; a number were already calling to ask if such a facility was available. Because many of these older Finns were fluent only in Finnish, they had problems when they went into Canadian nursing homes where English was the main language. For this reason the management at that time was keeping them in the congregate wing in cases where they should have been moved.

The development management was also not satisfied with present nursing assistance to their congregate residents, a number of whom had physical limitations, including the use of a cane, walking aid, or wheelchair. Because most of the congregate residents had come when they already had physical problems and because most were 80 or over, there was a continual need for nursing assistance. In 1972 it had been met only by a doctor making regular visits every two weeks and by a visiting community nurse coming in occasionally to help a few patients. This nursing help was felt to be inadequate as the nurse only performed a few jobs, such as giving medications, and the nurse could only stay a short time due to a heavy work load; also, the nurse was not available evenings or weekends, and was too busy to get to adequately know patient needs. At that time, the development staff wished they could have their own nursing staff who regularly could take on these jobs; all they had was a personal aide they used as a sort of nurse's aide to those in wheelchairs and to persons with canes.

This situation was changed somewhat when the nursing unit was built in Burnaby. The persons with more serious illnesses in the congregate wing could now be moved to the society's own nursing unit, and several were. However, the visiting community nurse still is used for the remaining congregate residents as well as apartment residents.

In sum, by 1976 the society had a multilevel system, with a predominance of apartment units but also congregate units, which apartment residents could move into when their health declined, as happened with some each year, and nursing units, which other congregate or apartment residents could move to when the necessity called for such. The society concentrated on apartment units, building more of these, because that was where the main demand was, both in 1963 when they first built, and in 1974 when they added their second development. The management told us that people tried to avoid taking a congregate unit until they were so sick they could no longer possibly stay in the apartment; some of these elderly considered the congregate housing an institutional setting for sick elderly.

The apartment dwellers did have the security of having a congregate unit next to them and a nursing unit run by the same society fairly close. These residents could use the dining room when the need came up; one or two also used the community meals-on-wheels service.

The residents also had an activities program available for them to use. There were bingo games twice a week, exercise programs, choir practice, handicrafts. They had a sauna available to them several times a week, and many made use of it. They had an extensive library. Even with all this, as well as the teas, picnics, religious services (either there or, from 1974 on, in the sister development, with arranged bus service to the latter) there still is need for expansion. The manager in 1972 felt more recreational activities were needed for the congregate residents, who he considered too passive. He felt a recreational worker was needed as the manager had too many jobs to adequately cover recreation. He felt it should be a staff person as he thought such a setup worked better than bringing in community persons. He said some outside funding was badly needed to pay for such a person as the costs could not be charged to the rents. This manager also felt outside recreation was needed but his residents did not have the strength for lawn bowling. A swimming pool had been considered but seemed impractical.

This development was somewhat inaccessible to community activities as it was a half hour from downtown. There was a public transportation stop a block from the development, but the hill was steep, and in winter residents worried about the ice as well as waiting for a bus in the cold or rainy weather. There was a shopping center right down the hill. The bus running between the two developments was also used to take people shopping. A community program called "Step Out" also occasionally took residents on pleasure trips.

The apartment residents got out rather regularly but many of the congregate residents did not. Many of the latter had no immediate family that they visited or visited them regularly.

In sum, this is a pleasant development that offers multilevel care and a wide variety of activities. For elderly of Finnish origin it provides a sense of community, of belonging, of security. For the approximately 30 percent of the residents who are not Finnish, it is less attractive as they feel somewhat like outsiders.

CULLODEN COURT,
VANCOUVER, BRITISH COLUMBIA

Culloden Court, Vancouver, is a public housing project constructed in 1967 that had, at the time of the case study, one senior citizens building of 44 bachelor and one-bedroom apartment units, and a number of low-rise row buildings (none larger than 14 units) housing a total of 86 families. The buildings, which also included a recreation hall, were attractively shingled and blended in with the architecture of the main single-family dwellings in this residential area. The lawns were well attended and there were flower gardens. The neighborhood was a pleasant working- and lower-middle-class area between 20 and 30 minutes from downtown; on one side were working-class bungalows and on the other, larger houses with three to five bedrooms.

There was easy public transportation to the downtown area from the development. There was also good access to shopping and to churches and a community center. The community offered such services as homemaker, meals-on-wheels, and visiting nurse services, and one or two of the residents used some of these. The community also had ample senior citizens centers, libraries, and such. Several organizations, the Parks Board, and the British Columbia Old Age Pensioners, offered programs there.

The development itself did have both a separate recreational building with lounge space, and, in the senior citizen building, a small lounge on the second floor reserved for the elderly's use. There was a lobby-mailbox area and a laundry facility in the elderly's building. The building did not have an elevator to the second floor. Recreational staff at the time of the study was in terms of a city Parks Board part-time paraprofessional recreation worker who lived in one of the family units. The public housing authority (British Columbia Housing Management Commission) now houses the area manager for a number of projects in an area office at Culloden Court, but at the time of the study there was no on-site manager. An area community relations worker (a graduate social worker) is also housed there; she acts as an information and referral person and tries to stimulate use of community services and bring services to them, such as the recent flu vaccination program. She helps bring in outside assistance for the project's overall tenant association and stimulate youth programs, but she is not a recreation worker. She has helped keep the new senior group, New Horizons, active. There is also a resident caretaker who pays only $50 to live there and does some minor maintenance.

Eleven of the 68 elderly residents of the senior citizen building were interviewed, and their average age was 70. Only four of the 11 indicated "no physical incapacity" as their health condition. One was in a wheelchair but could keep house. Of these 11 households, five were married couples, one a widower, one a divorced man, and the rest widows. Half formerly lived in apartments in that area.

Residents got out to downtown areas or to visit friends, and also interacted with other residents of the building. Half of those interviewed visited at least weekly within the building and a number of residents had even worked out a daily check system among themselves. They had an active Tenants Association, which the families also belonged to.

The residents had ample indoor recreational space, both in the multipurpose recreational building, with its small kitchen, table tennis, pool, and card table areas, and to some degree in their second-floor lounge, although it was so small that it was not used much. There was an active recreation program. However, they lacked other facilities found in some specially designed apartment complexes for the elderly and, more important, they had to share these facilities with the project families, and especially their children.

While there was some degree of territorial division of the project area, the multipurpose recreational center was shared by both the elderly and the families. In addition, the elderly's building was so situated to be between the elementary school and the family buildings, so that children from the development crossed the yard of the elderly's building. The entrance to the multipurpose recreational building faced the senior citizen building, so that when teenagers loitered outside the recreational building, before or after events, they were again in or near the elderly's territory. At the time of the study, there was a lack of playground, such as an adventure playground, or sufficient recreational staff to work with the children, so that play was scattered and nondirected; much of the play tended to be in the paved area between the recreation center and the senior citizens building. Some elderly felt the children's noisy play and the teenagers late-night wanderings impinged on their rest. As the recreation worker said, there was a problem of "overexposure" to children. The steady diet of children playing, of teenagers loitering or having noisy parties at the recreation center annoyed the elderly. Some residents spoke of teenagers swearing, playing pool and poker, throwing rocks at their windows, and of minor vandalism. The families believed some of the elderly residents provoked the children, for example, by staring endlessly from their windows. Recently playground equipment has been added in an area away from the senior housing.

The families were also annoyed that the elderly dominated the Tenants Association and that the elderly felt the multipurpose recreational center was their exclusive property; the elderly did domi-

nate the association. Interestingly, these elderly also had resented
the fact that in the early days of the project, residents of the surrounding neighborhood had been invited by management to use the building.
They considered these neighbors intruders; some still came to the
British Columbia pensioners meetings and today many come to a variety of activities such as bingo, social events, outings, crafts and
lectures organized by a New Horizons Senior Community Club.

At the time of our visits the friction between the elderly and
the families was being reduced by the presence of a very part-time
Parks Board recreation worker who made a great effort to get cooperation between the two groups. This worker lived in the family part
of the project, but her work was mainly with the elderly, under the
direction of the local nearby community center. She instigated a
variety of daytime recreational activities for these seniors, including
Wednesday bingos, special events, tours, and dancing, and she took
on individual counseling. She also acted as an information and referral person and an emergency service for them. She acted as a
liaison with the off-site manager.

She helped the elderly understand the children's need for a recreational outlet, so that when interviewed, several spoke of the need
for a youth-recreational worker and an adventure playground. Some
of these elderly also developed a concern for provision of play equipment for the children, such as more toys and sports equipment. The
recreation worker got both groups, the elderly and the families, to
work together on the Tenants Association and to run youth programs.
She even did some shopping and cleaning for them on a volunteer
basis. She unfortunately is no longer doing this job but the present
community relations worker has helped in some of these ways. She
has nurtured the New Horizons Senior Club as well as the Tenant Association for all tenants.

These elderly still would have preferred a separate recreation
area of their own, larger than their small unusable building lounge.
And, like all our interviewed elderly residents across Canada, most
preferred to be both in a development that did not have families and
in an area that was not mainly family dwellings. The Culloden Court
residents certainly had a better situation than the many elderly public
housing tenants who are in predominantly family buildings, with maybe
one elderly resident per floor, or in buildings where one floor of 11
units is for the elderly, as in a White Plains, New York, public housing project.

Having a separate building in a project that includes family
housing may not be enough. If such a project is planned, great effort
must be made to isolate the elderly from the families. Some architects have designed barriers between the two types of housing or developed unique ways by which the elderly can see the children, such

as in a nursery school, but not be part of the scene or bothered by the noise. One must be cautious in such planning, though. The British Columbia Housing Management Commission told one of our staff at the time of the study that they were now avoiding building mixed senior citizens and families developments.

10

NURSING HOMES AS RESIDENCE
AND/OR HEALTH FACILITY
Ilse J. Volinn

Nursing homes represent one dimension within the potential continuum of housing for the elderly. As a health care facility, nursing homes function as a sector of the health care system and occasionally are the point of entry into that system.

The concept of "system" as applied by cybernetics appears useful in the context of the following discussion. John D. O'Donahue,[1] in his analysis of health manpower, graphically shows how a system represents a whole, composed of identifiable parts that are interrelated through means of communication. In addition to the multiple relationships within the overall health care system, strong ties exist with the educational, the economic, the political institutions, and diverse population factors.

Facilities, services, and patients can be identified as the major components of the health care system.

Although the above linkage is ever present, the theoretical framework concerned with institutional behavior supplies the unifying component for the complex network of geriatric care for the aged.

A CONCEPTUAL FRAMEWORK FOR THE ANALYSIS
OF NURSING HOMES: NURSING
HOMES AS TOTAL INSTITUTIONS

Erving Goffman's[2] conceptualization of "total institutions" places the focus on those characteristics they have in common. By considering nursing homes as a subcategory of total institutions, the overall conceptualization can be applied to their analysis. The identification of common features becomes a possible explanation of functional reasons. Such an approach reaches beyond the praise or blame of specific

245

individuals. An underlying structural design is applicable to problems and issues of total institutions.

Total institutions are best described by their all-encompassing character. People are moved in blocks. Individuals sleep, eat, and play with the same participants, in the same institutional setting, with no role differentiation. The preinstitutionalized way of life is not taken for granted and even ignored. A dispossession of preadmission social roles has taken place. The barriers between patients and the outer world seem insurmountable. A feeling of isolation is created. That is further strengthened through a lack of communication between patients and the outer world. Control of communication is one of the functions assigned to institutional personnel. All aspects of daily living—eating, sleeping, washing, toileting—previously subject to self-regulation are controlled and judged by the staff. Many private aspects of life have become public. Traditional customs such as food preference are ignored and replaced by unfamiliar substitution. Total institutions have processes of mortification in common—loss of adult autonomy and of bodily comfort. Restrictions are rationalized by the effort to manage daily activities of a large number of persons in a limited space, with the smallest possible expenditure of resources.

Long-Term Care Facilities: Definitions, Characteristics, Distribution

There is no uniform definition for nursing homes and long-term care institutions. Their complexity and dynamics make their study particularly interesting and challenging.

The lack of uniform definitions and of clearly defined goals has been described in various ways. John Madge[3] quotes Peter Townsend (The Last Refuge) in urging a clarification of the following issues:

1. Are long-term care facilities a permanent refuge for infirm persons who are not in need of continuous nursing care?
2. Are they a temporary arrangement for persons recovering from acute episodes of illness?
3. Are they a refuge for persons who need comprehensive care?
4. Are they a haven for older persons who need primarily "protected housing?"

Madge[4] suggests the establishment of various kinds of accommodations on a single site with a great overall degree of flexibility.

Part of the National Health Survey program, conducted by the National Center of Health Statistics (NCHS), are the studies on long-term care facilities; publication of the data occurs periodically, with date of data gathering and date of publication, always indicated on the title page, usually showing a lapse of about two years. The data include information on the patient population and institutional characteristics such as ownership, size, geographic location, cost factors, and data relative to personnel employed.

The first survey in that series, referred to as Resident Places Survey 1, or RPS1[5] provides definitions for long-term care facilities. Later publications continue with the same definitions. Definitional criteria are (1) the number of persons receiving nursing care during the previous seven days; (2) the determination of medications and treatment administered in accordance with physicians' orders; (3) whether or not there is supervision over medication that may be self-administered; (4) the number of specified personal services routinely provided, such as help with bathing, eating, walking, or dressing; (5) presence or absence of nurses on the staff.

Congregate living facilities are considered long-term care institutions if they have at least three beds and routinely provide some level of nursing and/or personal care. Three categories of such facilities were defined, as follows:

1. Nursing care homes represent the highest level of health care—50 percent or more of the residents receive nursing care, which is provided either by registered nurses (RNs) or licensed practical nurses (LPNs). Nursing care refers to such procedures as administering of hypodermic and intravenous injections, catheterization, and oxygen therapy. Nursing care homes represent 63 percent of all the long-term care facilities, 78 percent of the beds, and 78 percent of the residents.

2. Personal care-with-nursing homes presuppose that (a) over 50 percent of the residents receive nursing care, although neither RNs nor LPNs are on the staff; or (b) less than 50 percent of the residents receive nursing care but one or both of the following conditions are met: medication is administered according to physicians' orders and/or there is supervision over self-medication; or (c) three or more personal services are provided. Personal care-with-nursing homes represent 21 percent of the facilities, 17 percent of the beds, and 17 percent of the residents.

3. Personal care homes represent the lowest level of long-term health care. The residents routinely receive personal care, including supervision of medication and treatment. Personal care homes represent 17 percent of the facilities, 5 percent of the beds, and 5 percent of the residents.

An estimated 18,391 long-term care facilities within the United States were reported;[6] further details are reflected in Table 10.1.

Definitions Based on Certification of Nursing Homes

Between the passage of Title XVIII and Title XIX of the Social Security Act in 1965 and the unification of the two separate nursing home certification programs in 1972, the following categorization and terminology was applied: (1) extended care facility (ECF)—for institutions certified by Medicare; (2) skilled nursing facility (SNF)—certified by Medicaid; (3) intermediate care facility (ICF)—certified by Medicaid; (4) facilities that were not certified by either Medicare or Medicaid but were providing some level of nursing care.[7]

Some facilities were certified under either Medicare or Medicaid and others held both certifications. Some homes were certified to participate in the Medicaid program as a skilled nursing home and as an intermediate care facility.

In order to qualify for reimbursement through the Title XVIII program, a nursing home has to be certified. The conditions are specified by the Social Security Administration.[8] The regulations refer to patient care policies concerning admission, transfer and discharge, personnel policies, and to the physical environment of the facility. Administrative management procedures are also specified. In summary, an ECF has to be in compliance with state and local licensing laws as well as with federal regulations.

An NCHS survey[9] conducted prior to the actual implementation of the unification of certification standards includes the information that 77 percent of the long-term care facilities were certified by Medicare, by Medicaid, or by both programs. Those without certification were the smallest facilities, averaging 45 beds. The national estimate of the distribution of facilities and residents at the time of that survey (August 1973 to April 1974) was 157,000 nursing homes, 1,174,800 beds, and 1,075,800 residents.

In 1972 Congress created unified standards and regulations governing skilled nursing facilities under Title XVIII and Title XIX. Skilled nursing homes, infirmary sections of homes for the aged, and skilled nursing home wings in hospitals are included in the following definition.

A skilled nursing facility is:

a specially qualified facility which has the staff and equipment to provide skilled nursing care and rehabilitation services as well as other related health services. Skilled nursing care is under the supervision of licensed nursing personnel. Skilled rehabilitation services may include physical therapy performed by or under the supervision of professional therapists. Nursing and rehabilitation services must be under the general direction of a doctor.

TABLE 10.1

Long-Term Care Institutions, by Type of Service, Ownership, and
Number of Beds

Institution	Type of Service	Type of Ownership	Number of Beds
Nursing care			
Number	11,576	—	—
Percent	62.9	—	—
Personal care with nursing			
Number	3,768	—	—
Percent	20.5	—	—
Personal care			
Number	3,047	—	—
Percent	16.6	—	—
Proprietary			
Number	—	14,161	—
Percent	—	77.0	—
Nonprofit			
Number	—	2,847	—
Percent	—	15.5	—
Government			
Number	—	1,383	—
Percent	—	7.5	—
Under 30 beds			
Number	—	—	8,100
Percent	—	—	44.0
30–49 beds			
Number	—	—	3,574
Percent	—	—	19.4
50–99 beds			
Number	—	—	4,573
Percent	—	—	24.9
Over 100 beds			
Number	—	—	2,144
Percent	—	—	11.7

Source: National Center for Health Statistics, Selected Characteristics of Nursing Homes for the Aged and Chronically Ill (Washington, D.C.: Department of Health, Education and Welfare, Health Services and Mental Health Administration, June–August 1974).

Skilled nursing and rehabilitation services have to be
needed on a daily continuous and not on an occasional
basis.[10]

In 1975 the regulations for skilled nursing facilities were altered
again. Two significant differences from the old extended care definitions are as follows: "Patients who require skilled rehabilitation
services in an institution are covered even though they may not need
skilled nursing services . . . [and] persons who need a variety of
services which individually may be unskilled but which considered in
the aggregate require management by skilled nursing personnel may
be found to need skilled nursing facility services."[11]

The Historical Development of Long-Term Care

Originally, homes for the aged were established by churches
and religious orders to care for the elderly sector of the population
considered as physically and economically incapable to function independently. Dorothea Jaeger and Leo W. Simmons[12] describe these
patients as highly homogeneous relative to age, nationality, ethnic
background, and religion.

Gradually, the population utilizing long-term care facilities
changed. Persons 65 years and older had numerically become a
more predominant sector of the total population. Urbanization and
industrialization had resulted in urban concentrations of patients,
services, and facilities. The extended family increasingly became a
nuclear family. The 1935 Social Security legislation provided older
people with additional funds. Based on a combination of these factors,
nursing homes were not only used by persons with very limited means
but also by those who could afford to pay for institutional care.

Charles J. Karcher and Leonard L. Linden[13] give one of the
many possible interpretations of these trends: the family as a social
institution had ceased to be a self-sufficient unit; family participation
in the care of older persons had decreased; the number of members
in a family had become smaller.

The trend to institutionalize older persons increased; within the
family unit they had lost their formerly prescribed social roles. The
sick role provided a meaningful substitution for that loss. In many
cases that sick role was inappropriate and resulted in institutionalization of many financially able persons with families, who realistically
did not require nursing care and could be classified as healthy aged.

Goffman[14] characterized nursing home patients as basically
harmless to society but incapable of managing without help.

Legislation and Congressional Committees

The impact of changes in population compositions, social values, and health behavior became increasingly apparent. Dissatisfaction with the modes of health care delivery has been growing. Legislative action is a manifestation of the effort to change existing institutions. Legislative actions and congressional committee activities demonstrate the changing trends in long-term care.

The Hospital Survey and Construction Act, later known as the Hill-Burton Program, was enacted in 1946. It was a response to the need for replacement of many hospitals and long-term care facilities that had become obsolete during World War II. That time represented a moratorium in the building of community-based health facilities.

The act specified financial assistance for construction. The federal government and local communities shared the responsibilities for implementation of the act. An important aspect of that legislation was the planning component, which paved the way for further efforts to coordinate the delivery of health care. Interrelationships between health facilities had to be demonstrated. Criteria for the assessment of the physical plants were formulated. Planning regions within state boundaries were delineated. James D. Hepner and Donna M. Hepner[15] consider that act as the basis for such planning legislation as the Regional Medical Program (RMP) and the Comprehensive Health Planning Act (CHP).

The 1965 legislation establishing Medicare and Medicaid drastically increased the demand for long-term care facilities. A large number of proprietary nursing homes were built during the following years, and many establishments were vastly enlarged.

Medicare and Medicaid Legislation

Public Law (PL) 89-97 established Medicare and Medicaid[16] under Title XVIII and Title XIX of the Social Security Act. That legislation was passed by Congress in 1965.

Medicare is a health insurance program administered by the Bureau of Health Insurance, Social Security Administration (SSI), of the U.S. Department of Health, Education and Welfare (HEW). The medical and institutional bills for insured persons are paid with money from trust funds, since the program is financed by payroll contributions.

The program helps to pay for hospital inpatient care, aftercare in skilled nursing homes, home care provided by a home health agency, and for such services as diagnostic laboratory tests, transportation by ambulance, and physical therapy. Kidney dialysis and transplant services are also included in the insurance coverage.

Claimants receive the benefits as a matter of right. The coverage includes persons 65 years and older and some disabled persons who have been entitled to social security disability payments for at least two consecutive years.

Medicare does not cover the cost of so-called custodial care, including assistance in activities of daily living, such as eating, walking, bathing, and dressing. The primary emphasis is on care that requires professional skills and training.

A basis for reimbursement is a minimum of three days as a hospital inpatient and a medical diagnosis that represents the same episode of illness as that in existence at the time of hospital admission. The overall focus is on posthospital care. Medicare benefits cover only such care as rendered by a certified nursing home. Certification is obtained by demonstrating compliance with federal regulations directed to accomplish a specified level of quality of care. The federal program of Medicare is the same all over the United States.

Medicaid (Title XIX of the Social Security Act) is a welfare program.[17] Money from federal, state, and local taxes pay medical bills for eligible persons. The program is administered by state government, with federal guidelines. The federal agency carrying the responsibility is the Medical Services Administration, Social and Rehabilitation Services, of HEW. The program is financed by federal and state governments. Unlike Medicare, it is not uniform throughout the United States. Except for mandatory services, the amount, scope, and duration of services, as well as eligibility regulations and benefits, vary from state to state.

Medicaid is a federal grant-in-aid program in which the federal government pays 50-83 percent of the costs incurred by the state in providing medical assistance.

Eligibility to Title XIX benefits is tied into the federal welfare categories and application processes. Services, including nursing home care, are provided for that sector of the population falling within a specified category of low income. Many aged persons are included in that definition.

The survey and certification process of long-term care facilities is basically a state responsibility. The regional director of HEW assures consistency of policy interpretation.

In December 1971, Congress authorized the participation of intermediate care facilities in Medicaid programs (PL 92-223).

Medicare and Medicaid Uniform Standards

PL 92-603, signed October 30, 1972, mandated a single set of nursing home standards. The federal regulations were published by HEW in January 1974. They provide the mechanism for inspecting and certifying nursing homes receiving federal funds.

Congressional Hearings—the Moss Reports

Senator Frank E. Moss of Utah is (at this writing) the chairman of the Subcommittee on Long Term Care, of the Special Committee on Aging. The subcommittee's hearings in 1963, 1964, and 1965[18] led to the Moss Amendments of 1976, which brought about major nursing home reforms.

The Moss Amendments of 1967 were tailored to meet the most significant problems that had been disclosed during the subcommittee hearings. They included provisions for home health services as an alternate to nursing home care, emphasis on detailed record keeping relative to all services, and increased efforts to define requirements for "sufficient nursing and auxiliary personnel."

The entire findings[19] of the subcommittee hearings will be contained in a series of 12 volumes, composed of the introductory report and 11 supporting papers. As of this writing (May 1976), seven supporting papers have been published; the others are forthcoming. Summaries of the forthcoming supporting papers, as well as major points of the published volumes, are contained in each of the publications.

Medicaid[20] currently pays about 60 percent of the nation's nursing home bills, and Medicare another 7 percent. Medicaid makes up the difference between social security benefits of retired persons and the cost of nursing home care. Because of the lack of a coherent policy on clearly defined goals and methods, many persons are left without necessary care. Such action could be avoided by viable home health care and other supportive services.

PL 92-603 had little effect on either eligibility or level of care. It specified that the merger of Medicaid and Medicare standards should, in case of former discrepancies, maintain those standards that, in prior certification regulations, had specified higher levels of care. In spite of these directives, new standards were formulated by HEW. These were too vague for enforcement.

On August 1, 1971, then President Nixon announced an eight-point plan to improve nursing homes. He proposed:

1. Federal training for nursing home inspectors.
2. New HEW positions to aid enforcement of regulations.
3. Federal reimbursement for 100 percent of the cost of state inspections of nursing homes.
4. Centralization of enforcement activities in one HEW office.
5. Short-term training programs for nursing personnel.
6. Authorization for HEW to assist in state investigations of consumer complaints.

7. Comprehensive study of long-term care by HEW to develop rec-
   comendations for action.
8. Recommendation to cut off federal Medicare and Medicaid funds to
   those facilities that did not meet the specified standards.

Although five ombudsman units were funded in 1972, no legislative action was taken to require each state to set up such a program.

Many examples[21] of negligence, fire hazards, and food poison-
ing in nursing homes were discovered. Such evidence of substandard
care demonstrates the need for extensive changes in the system of
long-term care.

Nursing home patients[22] take an average of 4.2 different medications per day, according to a 1975 report. Later studies estimate
that average to be 7.0. In 1972, drugs accounted for 10 percent of
all nursing home expenditures. Tranquilizers constitute almost 20
percent of all drugs. A 20-40 percent error rate is estimated, and
the overall misuse has been documented. The main contributing factor is the employment of untrained aides and orderlies. Frequent
kickbacks connected with drug purchases have been discovered.

Current trends[23] in medical education are largely responsible
for the shortcomings in long-term care. A 1971 survey showed that
geriatrics as a specialty had not been established in any of the medical schools. In 1974, 13 schools provided a curriculum in geriatrics,
and 26 schools placed interns, residents, or students in nursing homes
for the fulfillment of their academic requirements.

The underreporting of infectious diseases in nursing homes is
an additional shortcoming of the lack of medical care. About 80-90
percent[24] of the care in nursing homes is provided by untrained and
unlicensed personnel. They are overworked and underpaid. Federal
standards for skilled nursing facilities call for one registered nurse
during the day shifts. Intermediate care facilities are required to
employ one licensed practical nurse on day shift. The remaining
long-term care facilities are not required to have any licensed nursing staff at all.

Ratios between nurses and patients are not specified in any of
the federal regulations. Nursing home staffs lack medical support
and continuous contact with professionals, as is the case in hospital
settings. Geriatrics as a specialty in schools of nursing is a rarity.

Some 7,200[25] of the nation's 23,000 long-term care facilities
do not participate in federal programs and therefore meet only such
standards as are promulgated by the state. In 1971, 4,800 nursing
home fires were reported. A General Accounting Office (GAO) study
in 1974 indicated that 72 percent of the nation's nursing homes have
one or more major fire deficiencies; 59 percent of SNFs were certified with deficiencies, and 60 percent of ICFs do not comply with

existing standards. The Life Safety Codes of the National Fire Protection Association are frequently not enforced, and their interpretation by inspecting surveyors is not uniform.

Supporting Paper 6[26] of the Moss reports is entitled What Can
Be Done in Nursing Homes: Positive Aspects in Long Term Care.
It conveys the belief that physical and mental problems of the elderly
are, to a substantial degree, preventable and frequently reversible.
The importance of increasing education for nursing home administrators is stressed. Innovative techniques of long-term care are emphasized. Among these is reality orientation, sensory training, and
remotivation to participate in activities. Points for improved physical structure of the facilities specify means for better care as well
as greater comfort. Participation in peer review programs and support of ombudsman projects are stressed. Information relative to
the forthcoming Moss reports is based on the summaries included
in Supporting Paper 6.

Among the positive aspects of nursing home care has been the
executive order[27] of then President Nixon to establish an ombudsman
program. Responses ranged from the publication of nursing home
directories with rating systems to peer reviews and the establishment
of a "cool line" in Chicago, which provides a telephone number to
voice complaints.

Thousands of elderly patients[28] have been transferred from
state mental institutions to nursing homes. This procedure substi-
tutes federal money for state dollars. Two and one-half million elderly are going without the mental health services they need. Nursing homes are ill equipped to meet their needs. They lack psychiatric
services, do not make plans for psychological rehabilitation, and
are not included in followup procedures from state hospitals. Between
1969 and 1974, 56 percent of the elderly inmates of state hospitals
were returned to the community. The physically infirm and the men-
tally impaired are living in close proximity in most nursing homes.
Deleterious effects are a consequence.

Recommendations for improvement include reimbursement
mechanisms for outpatient psychiatric care, effective professional
preadmission screening procedures, and specifications for followup
care for post-mental hospital patients.

Minorities[29] have limited access to nursing homes. Only 4
percent of the one million nursing home patients represent ethnic
minorities, even though their health needs are greater than that of
the rest of the population. Cost, lack of information about Medicaid,
discrimination, language barriers (particularly for Spanish-speaking
persons and Japanese-Americans), rural isolation, and cultural problems are the main causes for the imbalance.

It was found that 106 publicly held corporations[30] controlled
18 percent of the nursing home industry's beds and accounted for
one-third of the industry's $3.2 billion in revenue.

The last two papers of the Moss series will consist of a com-
pendium of statements issued by national organizations and administration spokesmen and the final report by the subcommittee.

Toward Quality Care of the Aged:
Professional Nurses Speak

The American Nurses Association, as part of a project called
"Nursing and Long Term Care: Toward Quality Care for the Aging,"
issued a report in 1975.[31] The findings include discussions of current institutional shortcomings as well as suggestions to rectify the
barriers to optimum care for the elderly.

The current Medicare reimbursement system encourages the
overuse of institutions. A solution could be found in the broadening
of coverage, with greater emphasis on a wide range of services.
Identification of appropriate settings for each potential resident
should be a focus. Reimbursement under the current federal system
of patient classifications is based on the number of hours provided
by professional personnel. A more appropriate criterion would be
the assessment of patients' need for specified services. The changing
health status should be reflected by a flexible classification system.

Current Medicare regulations deny skilled nursing care for the
chronically ill, low-income persons because admission to an SNF
is based on an episode of acute illness. Medicare benefits are dis-
continued when a patient's condition has become stabilized. Interrup-
tion of treatment follows. The consequences are serious effects on
the patient's health.

Standards for Long-Term Health Care

The National Health Planning Resources and Development Act
of 1974 (PL 93-641)[32] requires that health planning agencies review
all institutional health services on a periodic basis. An assessment
of their availability, accessibility, appropriateness, and adequacy
is mandated. Their regulatory and review authority makes the construction of operational criteria and standards imperative.

The Health Care Services Criteria Project at the University of
Washington[33] is a response to the legislative challenge. The project
formulated that the following essential characteristics of the operational standards and criteria should:

1. be in the public interest;
2. reflect current and accurate technical, clinical, epidemiological, and therapeutic knowledge relevant to specific services;
3. make health objectives and health problems explicit;
4. consider the variability and complexity of health services;
5. be measurable;
6. specify the factual basis composing criteria;
7. allow for a range of success and failure;
8. be applicable to the health planning review process;
9. allow for local approaches;
10. reflect community values and goals;
11. be understandable to laymen;
12. encourage citizen participation;
13. precede the considerations of the planning body;
14. consider money, personnel, and facility resources that would be required to implement the criteria and standards.

Standards for different levels of care were developed. Long-term care is seen as a continuum of inpatient and outpatient services. Adequate care refers to the compatibility of different types of health services, including the degree of comprehensiveness and continuity of care. A prerequisite is the accurate and current knowledge relative to the technology of specific services. Treatment goals should be related to clinical, epidemiological, and therapeutic aspects of a treatment program. The need for care provided by a spectrum of health professionals should be determined through a process of evaluating the patient's health status. This also applies to the assessment, periodicity, and frequency of medical visits; levels of nursing care; and training in activities of daily living (ALD). The criteria for long-term health care will be applied to the measurement of a range of relative success and failure of long-term care services.

PERSONNEL EMPLOYED IN NURSING HOMES

Professional Roles

Anselm Strauss[34] elaborates on the role of personnel in long-term care facilities. Health professionals should be responsible for the family of patients, in addition to the patients. They also should be expected to put effort into the establishment of community ties.

By shifting the emphasis from specific tasks to an understanding of the sick person as a whole, including the physical and social environment, a wide range of services becomes imperative, such as social and psychological counseling, overall coordination of health care, and consumer advocacy. The services would best be delivered by a team, with the patients as active participants in the management of their illness. Strauss proposes that training necessarily would have to prepare the professionals for the newly established goals of long-term care. These skills would have to be in addition to the knowledge of technical aids and equipment, medical intervention, and daily maintenance of the patients.

Distribution of Personnel

National statistics provide an overview of personnel employed in long-term care facilities. Nursing and nursing home administration will be discussed below in some detail. Since space does not allow the same coverage for all the health professionals who contribute to long-term, institutionalized care, some omissions are necessary.

The NCHS reports that the total number of nursing home employees is 553,879.[35] The nursing staff represented 59.7 percent. The distribution of each of the three categories of nursing personnel expresses relative levels of preparatory training—7.7 percent were registered nurses; 8.7 percent, licensed practical nurses; and 43.3 percent, nurse's aides. Other professional and technical personnel comprised 10.5 percent. That category includes dieticians, physical therapists, occupational therapists, speech therapists, and recreation therapists. "Other staff," which includes administrators, represented 4.9 percent. Employees categorized as "non-professional staff" represented 29.8 percent. The average staffing pattern was six full-time equivalent (FTE) employees for every ten residents.

Nursing Home Administrators

The 1967 amendment to Title XIX (Medicaid) of the Social Security Act required all states and other jurisdictions participating in Medicaid to license by waiver or examination all nursing home administrators by July 1, 1970. Federal guidelines, among other standards, proposed that applicants hold a high school diploma or equivalent and pass an approved course of study in nursing home administration. In proper time sequence, increase of academic training for that position is proposed, from two years of college in 1975, to bachelor's degree in 1980, to master's degree in 1985. Possible substitution of practical experience in nursing home administration for formal schooling is spelled out.

An NCHS nationwide survey[36] showed that 21 percent of the nursing home administrators had less than twelfth-grade schooling, and

the remaining 79 percent had twelfth-grade schooling at least, sometimes more. The majority, 71 percent, had four years or more of
employment. The median was eight years of employment. Regional
differences were discerned. In the South and West there were more
respondents who had worked less than four years as administrators
than in other parts of the country. Of all the administrators, 90 percent had no prior experience as hospital administrators. Long working hours are a characteristic of the profession, with a mean of 57
hours per week. Those self-employed worked longer hours than those
administrators who were employees. Administrators in small facilities (less than 30 beds) worked longer hours than those in larger
homes.

    Before reporting on a survey that was conducted in the state of
Washington, it is relevant to refer to the rules and regulations of the
Board of Examiners of the nursing home administrators in the state
of Washington. During the 1969-70 session, Washington State legis-
lators decreed that it should be mandatory for all persons operating
a nursing home to be licensed as provided in Chapter 18.52 of the state
law. The intent of the Nursing Home Administrators Practice Act
was to "establish and provide for the enforcement of standards for
the licensing of nursing home administrators."[37] The governor
appointed the state Board of Examiners, composed of nine members.
Qualifications for licensees were formulated. The Nursing Home Administrators Practice Act also contains specifications on such matters
as provisional licenses, licensing duties and responsibilities, processing of complaints, and revocation of license.

    The 1971 survey of nursing home administrators licensed in
the state of Washington[38] identified variations in the professional
role of nursing home administrators: 69 percent were administrators
or assistants, regional executives, assistant directors, or presidents
of corporations; 25 percent were owners, coowners, or partners; 6
percent assumed more than one professional role. Nursing home administration was combined with hospital administration, retirement
home administration, supervision of nursing services, or the position
of the institution's controller or secretary. Administrators in charge
of a single nursing home represented 82.1 percent; 7.1 percent operated two homes; 7.9 percent were in charge of three to five facilities;
and the remaining 2.9 percent were administrators of six or more
homes (the largest number of homes administered by one person was
21).

    Fifty-eight percent of the respondents were men. The majority
of all administrators, 62 percent, were between the ages of 36 and
55. Forty-two percent had pursued some post-high school education;
33 percent had earned a baccalaureate or higher degree; 22 percent
were high school graduates; and 4 percent had less than a high school

education. Many major fields of training were identified, such as education, home economics, pharmacy, dentistry, psychology, history, religion and the ministry, political science, medicine, and hospital and hotel administration. The two major fields were nursing/nursing education (62 out of 212 respondents) and business administration (32 out of 212 respondents). Thirty-nine percent of the respondents held an additional license, certification, or registration, in fields such as nursing (RN, LPN), medicine (MD, DO), accounting (CPA), or real estate.

Nurses as Nursing Home Administrators

The trend for professional nurses to function as nursing home administrators and/or supervisors is increasing. It was in recognition of this fact that a national conference for nursing home administrators and directors was called for August 1-2, 1974.[39] The stated purpose was to "provide direction in approaches to improve quality of care for the aged in nursing homes." The conference resulted in identification of the following problem areas that deter delivery of quality nursing care: (1) health care providers' lack of interest in nursing home care; (2) barriers to continuity of care; (3) lack of clarity concerning the role of the nurse-administrator in nursing homes. Recommendations to the ANA were formulated and areas for assistance by the professional association were specified.

Professional Nurses in Nursing Homes

The ANA[40] reported that 65,235 out of 815,000 professional nurses were employed in nursing homes. A similar distribution was found in the 1971 study of professional nurses in the state of Washington.[41] A comparison with earlier surveys showed that employment of professional nurses in nursing homes had been increasing. In 1975, 6.6 percent of the RNs licensed and residing in the state of Washington reported employment in nursing homes. This rose to 7.0 percent in 1961; 8.9 percent in 1969; and 9.4 percent in 1970. It is important to consider the major clinical and/or practice area for health professionals. The 1971 study[42] showed that 10.8 percent of a total of 10,636 professional nurses licensed and residing in the state of Washington in 1970 reported geriatric nursing as their field of specialization. Of these geriatric specialists, 74.8 percent were employed in nursing homes.

The primary work function of nurses employed in nursing homes in the state of Washington was explored. Table 10.2 shows the distribution. It can be seen that only 29 percent of the respondents per-

TABLE 10.2

Registered Nurses Residing in the State of Washington, by Type of
Position in Nursing Homes, 1970

Position	Number	Percent
Administrator	60	5.0
Supervisor	278	23.2
Head nurse	413	34.4
General duty	346	28.9
Other	102	8.5
Total	1,199	100.0

Source: Ilse J. Volinn, "Professional Nurses in Washington
State. A Comparison: 1970-1969-1961-1957," mimeographed
(Olympia, Wash.: State Department of Social and Health Services,
June 1971).

TABLE 10.3

Basic Nursing Education, by Nursing Home and Hospital Employment
of Registered Nurses Residing in the State of Washington, 1970

Education	Nursing Homes		Hospitals	
	Number	Percent	Number	Percent
Diploma	974	86.2	5,770	76.7
Associate degree	44	3.9	604	8.0
Baccalaureate or higher degree	112	9.9	1,154	15.3
Total	1,130	100.0	7,528	100.0

Source: Ilse J. Volinn, "Professional Nurses in Washington
State. A Comparison: 1970-1969-1961-1957," mimeographed (Olympia, Wash.: State Department of Social and Health Services, June
1971).

formed general nursing duties. The frequently heard comment that
the primary function of professional nurses in nursing homes is on
the administrative level is substantiated.

The three avenues of preparatory training to become a professional nurse are the diploma program, associate degree (AA), and

baccalaureate or higher degree. Hospital diploma programs, most popular in the past, are gradually phasing out. It can be seen in Table 10.3 that 86 percent of the registered nurses employed in nursing homes in the state of Washington held nursing diplomas.

A possible explanation of the differences in educational training might lie in the fact that nurses employed in nursing homes on the whole are older than those working in hospitals; at least this was found to be true in the state of Washington survey. Hospital or diploma schools were the usual course of training until the creation of community colleges and increased emphasis on baccalaureate degrees.

Nursing has become professionalized, and many members of the profession give vivid expressions to evolving functions and goals in long-term care. Doris R. Schwartz[43] emphasizes that a patient population characterized by hopelessness, helplessness, and lack of prestige presents a real challenge to the nursing profession. That challenge can be met, among others, by striving for continuity of care, prevention of progressive depersonalization, and routinization of services.

Practical Nurses

An NCHS survey in 1968[44] reports a total of 48,137 LPNs em ployed in nursing homes. Of these, 77 percent were full-time employees and the rest worked part time. The smaller the facility, the larger is the percentage of LPNs. Nursing home employment represents 13 percent of all employment settings for LPNs.

A survey[45] conducted in the state of Washington in 1969 provides further data concerning LPNs employed in nursing homes. Of those licensed and living in the state of Washington, 843 LPNs (16.3 percent) reported employment in nursing homes; 67.1 percent worked full time and 32.9 percent part time. This represents a lower percentage of full-time employment than that in hospitals or physicians' offices. The primary work function in nursing homes is reported in Table 10.4.

LPNs working in nursing homes have longer work experience than those employed in other settings. While 37 percent had been active as LPNs for over ten years, only 24 percent of hospital-based OPNs had such extended occupational experience. One-third of the LPNs employed in the state of Washington nursing homes were aged 55 years or older; one-fourth of the LPNs in hospitals fell in that age category.

TABLE 10.4

Licensed Practical Nurses, by Work Function in the State of
Washington, 1969

Work Function	Number	Percent
Direct patient care	521	61.8
Charge nurse, plus direct care	69	8.2
Administration/supervision, plus direct care	37	4.4
Charge nurse	130	15.4
Supervision and administration	52	6.2
Other	33	4.0
Total	842	100.0

Source: Ilse J. Volinn, "Practical Nurses Licensed in Washington State," mimeographed (Olympia, Wash.: State Department of
Social and Health Services, November 1969).

Nurse's Aides

Nurse's aides represent the most numerous category of nursing staff in long-term care facilities. They are not licensed, and
no preparatory training is required prior to employment. Their
orientation to the professional tasks consists of on-the-job training
and, possibly, supervision. The lack of such training prior to direct
contacts with patients is described by some of the participants in
Ralph Nader's study group[46] of nursing homes. One of the aides tells
how she was asked to follow a disoriented patient throughout the city
streets for hours. She did not know how to get the patient back to the
nursing home or even how to assist her in any way.

At times, the training provided to nonlicensed personnel is too
superficial to be functionary. Jaber F. Gubrium and Margaret
Ksanders[47] studied reality orientation procedures in nursing homes.
They found that the aides understood neither the goals nor the procedures of the potentially rehabilitative service. Their performance
was purely mechanical, without commitment to any goals. They
merely tried to pull off their roles as therapists, and they made deals
with the patients so that they responded in the expected manner.

PATIENTS IN LONG-TERM CARE FACILITIES

Of the civilian population aged 65 years and older,[48] 4 percent
reside in nursing and/or personal care homes. The number of ad-

missions to nursing homes in 1968 was 968,750. The total number of residents was 815,130. Of these, 89 percent were aged 65 years or older. The number of persons aged 60 and older in homes for the aged, and in nursing, convalescent and rest homes, as reported in the 1970 U.S. census, was 838,315.[49] In these facilities, 84 percent of the men and 93 percent of the women were aged 60 years and older. Fifty-four percent of the women, but only 39 percent of the men, were aged 80 years and over. In that age group, 96 percent of the institutionalized persons were Caucasians.

Information reported in the NCHS's Health in the Later Years[50] draws from four independent sources: its Division of Vital Statistics; Division of Health interview statistics; Division of Health examination statistics; and Division of Health resources statistics. It was found that approximately one-sixth of the nursing home residents are confined to bed at all times and one-fourth part of the time. About one-fourth cannot walk and one-sixth can walk only with assistance. One-half of all nursing home residents suffer from complete or partial mental deterioration. Thirty-four percent have a diagnosis of vascular lesions affecting the central nervous system; 28 percent suffer from diseases of the heart; 22 percent have arthritis and rheumatism; 22 percent have advanced senility.

A 1969 NCHS survey[51] reports that 29.9 percent of the nursing home residents stayed at the institution 12 months or less; 32 percent remained in a nursing home more than three years; and another third of the institutionalized population reported a length of stay over one year but less than three years.

In 1969,[52] about one-fifth of the patients received intensive care, while in 1964 only one-twentieth required such high-level care.

Dimensions of Chronic Illness

L. Mayo, chairman of the Commission on Chronic Illness, defined chronic illness as "all impairments or deviations from normal which have one or more of the following characteristics: they are permanent, leave residual disability, are caused by non-reversible pathological alteration, require special training of the patient for rehabilitation, may be expected to require a long period of supervision, observation or care."[53]

Strauss[54] explains that the usual goal in treating persons with acute disease is their cure, while for those with chronic diseases it is their care. Hospitals are health facilities for cure, nursing homes for care.

Approaches to chronic diseases include control of symptoms, management of regimen, and adjustment to changes in the course of

the disease. Psychosocial aspects include the patient's adjustment
to change in the course of the disease, worsening as well as improvement, and attempts to normalize life as much as possible.

In a nursing home, with patients suffering an average of 3.5
chronic diseases, the following considerations have to be multiplied
by the respective number of patients: (1) some regimens have to be
carried out twice or three times daily; (2) some are performed on a
strict schedule; (3) others are related to peak periods of symptoms;
(4) some create much discomfort to the patient; (5) others cause side
effects that have to be watched and/or managed.

Strauss[55] describes the implications of disease management,
such as unpredictability, periodic flareup, or sudden depletion of
energy. Disease management also includes a great variety of thera-
pies and unexpected physical and psychological side effects.

Death and Dying

Care provided to nursing home patients frequently refers to
terminal care. A study[56] conducted in 1968 compared patients in
four types of health facilities. The study showed that 15.2 percent
of the patients in extended care facilities and 28.2 percent of the patients in nursing homes without certification died at the facility. In
view of this fact, the issues of dying and of death are appropriate to
an overall discussion of nursing homes.

Barney G. Glaser and Strauss discuss the "status passage" of
death.[57] It includes decisions related to the following questions:

1. Where and how should it occur?
2. What kind of physical and psychological comfort should be provided?
3. Who is in charge of the overall management?
4. Who assists in carrying the emotional burden?

Questions of definition of death and the prolonging of life are further
considerations. The isolation in institutional settings is juxtaposed
to a home environment, which is the patient's domain.

Glaser and Strauss[58] refer to the management of the course of
death, as defined by the participants, patients, and social environment, as "dying trajectory," an individual's socially defined course
of dying. In some nursing homes, dying starts with the move to a
special room, symbolically marked off. Persons in nursing homes
frequently are already treated as socially and psychologically dead.
They are isolated from the community and, often, even from their
friends and family. In nursing homes, passagees do not exert control over their life style while in passage. That passage is traversed
in aggregate rather than collective fashion.

Two empirical studies describe death and dying in nursing homes from different perspectives. In Gubrium's "Death Worlds in a Nursing Home,"[59] death and dying are discussed in the context of "main events." Main events are characteristic of all formally organized social settings. Definitions of death and dying depend on the definer's position within the organizational structure. Patients are categorized already at the time of admission as residents, who are ambulatory, or as patients, who are bedridden. Patients and residents witness death and dying to different degrees, greatly depending on the physical layout of the facility. The fact that the barber shop is on the "patient floor" decreases the access for residents who want to avoid possible exposure to processes of dying. This inaccessibility is of great importance. Goffman[60] discusses the relationship of a self-image to the individual's access to "guise," such as an opportunity to go to a barber or beauty shop. The "decoration specialists" assist the institutionalized person to counteract the "personal defacement and stripping of usual appearance"; persons who are not patients witness but do not experience the "event."

Gubrium[61] describes how death worlds are behavioral definitions and ways of thinking about the process of dying and the final outcome of death. Differences could be observed between levels of institutional personnel. Floor staff are the most frequent witnesses of both process and outcome. They are responsible for "bed and body work." Gubrium found that they often treat the patients as socially and psychologically dead and discuss their conditions as if they were not present. The administrative and professional staff have little personal involvement and usually witness neither death nor dying. In contrast to the floor staff, they "manage" death scenes in terms of space, supervision, sequence of events, and formulation of policies. They hold high control over the patients, but death and dying are not part of their regular work.

Victor W. Marshall's "Organizational Features of Terminal Status Passage in Residential Facilities for the Aged"[62] describes two sociocultural milieu with different structures of time and different characteristics of the "dying career." In the nursing home, as in other total institutions, all aspects of life are carried out in the company of others, overall regimentation allowing for little differentiation. Death is highlighted. In contrast, the social structure of the retirement home facilitates community involvement and support. The shared perspective of the residents concerning the "status passage" brings about mutual support, lacking in a nursing home setting.

ARCHITECTURAL AND SOCIAL SPACE
IN NURSING HOMES

Architectural design is considered within the context of patients rather than facilities in order to focus on its impact on physical and psychological well-being.

R. Somner[63] represents the point of view that the physical environment is a molder of behavior. J. Weinberg[64] differentiates between internal and external stimuli to which human beings react. Environmental information is perceived differently by different individuals. The messages differ in relevancy. Physical disabilities, particularly of the sensory system, decrease decoding abilities. Such handicaps are further aggravated by sterile institutional environments, which only carry minimal information. Weinberg suggests a great emphasis on thermal, olfactory, aural, and visual stimuli for increased delineation of territorial messages.

Lynn E. McClannahan[65] differentiates between therapeutic and prosthetic living arrangements for nursing home residents. Both kinds of environments can modify "old behavior" and contribute to a decrease of social isolation created by diminishing physical and social skills. Environmental arrangements, prosthetic or therapeutic, should contribute to a patient's self-care skills, motor behavior, and verbal expressions. Examples of such aids are handrails, ramps, proper floor covering, adjustment of light switches, shelves and lamps, and convenient plumbing. Social abilities can be greatly increased by opportunities for verbal behavior in heterogenous social environments.

Madge[66] emphasizes the importance of such architectural details as the size and location of windows and their impact on personal privacy. Noise levels and the amount of lighting and heating are significant to the comfort of patients. Wide door openings are important for the convenience of persons who use prosthetic devices such as crutches, walkers, or wheelchairs. The design can increase the opportunity for ambulation and socialization and minimize the assumption of the sick role.

Accident prevention measures should have a high priority in order to prevent fires, burns, or falls. Structural aspects, considered from the psychological vantage point, include the application of the concepts of territoriality and social space.

Territoriality originated in biology and the study of animal behavior. L. A. Pastalan and D. H. Carson[67] applied it to the analysis of the behavior of older people. An important distinction is made between different kinds of privacy: solitude, intimacy, anonymity, and reserve.

Dean C. Jones[68] reports that spatial proximity of patients in a nursing home more often creates conflict situations than friendships.

Physical space can serve as a buffer. Heterogenous social environments can have similar effects. Psychological distance can be sub-
stituted for physical distance through emotional withdrawal. Such
mechanism should be considered when trying to interpret certain behavioral sets of long-term care patients.

Standards published by the Health Services Criteria Project[69]
in 1975 include architectural components of long-term care. The environment should represent a continuum with life in the community
and not be in sharp contrast with it. The health facility should,
through its physical design, provide for an encourage use by the
community. This would assist the patients in maintaining an awareness of community activities and would in turn create community
awareness of the facility and its patients. The stress invariably ex-
perienced by patients upon entry could be reduced by creating a rehabilitative rather than a custodial atmosphere.

Interrelationships between architectural environment and certain goals for the care of the elderly patient are important. In order
to provide many opportunities to make choices and decisions, the
architectural environment has to be flexible and adpative to change.
To make their own decisions is vital for self-confidence, and feelings
of dependency are damaging. All aspects of social and physical constraints should be minimized. It is advisable to designate specific
spaces for the training in daily living.

CONSUMER MOVEMENTS

The consumer movement brought about varied confrontations
between the providers and consumers of long-term care. The frac-
tionalization of federal responsibilities is described in Nader's report.[70] In 1971, six federal agencies among the 22 that deal with
health services were responsible for nursing homes. Three state
agencies, plus several local departments of government, took part
in licensing, inspections, and standards setting for long-term care
facilities. Responsibilities to supervise rehabilitative and restora-
tive programs for the patients and training of personnel lacked clear
lines of accountability.

The gap between government regulations and their actual implementation is discussed in "Public Interest Report No. 13: The
Nursing Home Cover-Up."[71] Section 2990 of PL 92-603 calls for
disclosure of inspection results of Medicare certified institutions.
The Social Security Administration was to make the results of Medicare participating facilities available to the public. The March 1973
HEW-SSA regulations failed to implement these requirements. Although summaries of inspection reports can be obtained, their lan-

guage is not understood by laypersons and there usually is a 90-day delay before obtaining them. The general public is not made aware of their right to ask for them.

"Public Interest Report No. 15: Is There an Ideal Form of Care of the Old?"[72] contains a discussion of the new concept of nursing homes. Suggested services include day care, disease detection, group and individual counseling, psychotherapy, outreach efforts, health education, and social services to patients and their families.

A Health Services Information Center was established in Washington, D.C., in 1974. The National Consumer League in Washington, D.C., published in 1974 New Help for the Consumer.[73] Shortly after the Freedom of Information Act was passed, the league started to issue digests of nursing home inspection reports and make suggestions concerning the choice of nursing homes. Among the suggested criteria were 2.25 hours of nursing care per patient, availability of medical and dental care, and nursing home meals adjusted to patients' convenience.

In 1971, then President Nixon established a listening post for nursing home complaints. After the initial flurry of complaints, the procedures became essentially inoperative. Seven demonstration projects have been awarded since June 1972. In 1973, the ombudsman demonstration projects[74] were transferred from the Public Health Service to the Administration on Aging. Since these projects have shown the effects of nursing home ombudsman activities, a program with broader operational bases was created. Each state is to develop a local complaints program. A full-time person was assigned to each state to provide leadership in the development of the program. That action became operative in 1976. The program thrust represents a local complaint mechanism for individuals and representatives of groups of concerned citizens. They function as advocates and become pressure groups for nursing home residents.

CASE STUDIES

Case 1

Case 1 is presented from the point of view of the family members of a nursing home patient. Background information: The location is the Pacific Northwest. Mr. and Mrs. A. had been living on a small farm outside the city limits of a town, population 10,054. They had been married for 52 years when Mr. A. suddenly died at age 87. Mrs. A., aged 84, could not comprehend or accept that loss. Night and day she wandered around the countryside and through the nearby town in search of her husband. Her family, who live in the Middle West, became increasingly concerned for her safety. Consecutively, three live-in companions were retained but were unable to control the unconsolable widow. Mrs. A.'s psychological condition deteriorated rapidly, although her physical condition seemed sound. The family, upon the physician's advice, decided to place her in a nursing home located near her former home. That choice was based on the assumption that a move to a midwestern metropolitan area would be traumatic. The selection of the specific nursing home was based on the consideration of similarity to current and past life style and familiarity with several of the patients in that particular facility.

The nursing home is a proprietary home with a bed capacity of 42. It is licensed as an ICF. Assurance of regular visits by the physician was given. The administrator's wife had training in geriatric nursing. In addition to informal visits by old friends, regular outings and visits were secured through a financial arrangement.

Mrs. A. did not socialize in the nursing home. She ate all meals in her room, which she shared with a blind, mute, paralyzed patient. She took pride in assisting her roommate. After several months she was moved to a different room, which she shared with a physically able, lively, retired nurse. Her behavior changed. She seemed to enjoy her meals in the dining room and participated in social activities.

Six months later, her daughter came for a visit, and with great concern observed that her mother had continuous difficulty in staying awake. Neither the physician nor the nurses offered any explanation. One month later, Mrs. A. was admitted to the local hospital. The family suspected improper drug administration, which had apparently brought about physical inactivity and further resulted in pneumonia. After about one week Mrs. A. was readmitted to the nursing home. Increased surveillance of drug administration was successfully stressed.

Several months later, Mrs. A. was admitted to a hospital for a bladder operation to control her ever increasing incontinence. The problematic aspect of that incidence was the degree of insensitivity to geriatric care demonstrated by hospital personnel—the surgeon, who had not anticipated that a postsurgical senile patient would remove her own catheter without his consent; the nurses, who served the meals without providing the patient with her dentures, which she was too timid to request. Recovered from the surgery, Mrs. A returned to the nursing home. Her physical and mental condition deteriorated further. An unannounced visit by her family found her resting comfortably in a private room, seemingly well attended by an attentive and gentle nursing staff.

The patient died at age 86. The primary cause of death was reported as cancer of the liver. The family is still wondering if other alternatives for her care would have been preferable.

Case 2

Case 2 presents the point of view of a patient, Ms. D., aged 83. Ms. D. had been professionally active. She was now living alone in an apartment a short distance from the place of her part-time employment. Periodically she took extensive trips. One day an accident occurred in her apartment. She slipped on her rug and was consequently taken to a hospital by ambulance. Her injury turned out to be minor, but a diagnosis of pneumonia, severe dehydration and malnutrition, as well as emphysema and a heart condition, prolonged her hospital stay. She was discharged to a nursing home after ten days.

It was a proprietary nursing home in a metropolitan area of the Pacific Northwest. The institution has a total of 128 beds, 29 of which are licensed as skilled nursing care beds. She was very disappointed when she discovered that her regular physician, connected with the health maintenance organization of which she is a member, could not attend her at the nursing home. A physician unknown to her was assigned to her. She had great difficulties in submitting to the institutional routine, as well as to such medical advice as to get out of bed and start to move about. Institutional food seemed unpalatable and bland to her, as she was used to a rather cosmopolitan cuisine. After several days she made the intellectual decision that full cooperation would be to her benefit. She asked to be helped to go to the general dining room and eat whatever was served to her. She at first was shocked by the experience of being surrounded by patients who were incoherent and demonstrated emotionally disturbed behavior, such as hiding her eating utensils. Soon she discovered two young persons, recovering from injuries, who were well educated and intelligent, and who were interesting company. She made it a point to sit near them during mealtime. Still, the behavior of the senile patients disturbed her. The nursing home staff offered to serve her meals in the lounge, but her newly found young friends objected to the loss of her interesting companionship. She was pleased to be accepted by those patients she considered desirable company.

She became increasingly involved in accelerating her training in ADL and made great efforts to become physically independent again. Her discharge was based on arrangements to maintain her in her own home. Several friends made a plan for meal preparation, shopping, transportation, and occasional outings. Ms. D. was discharged from the nursing home after a five-week stay. She returned to her apartment but is now preparing to move into a retirement home with nursing service available when necessary.

This chapter was designed to provide an overview to issues related to institutional care of the aged. It is important to view such care as part of a continuum of living arrangements, health care, community relations, economic management, and social and recreational activities.

Empirical data, research reports, and theories reported in this chapter hopefully will stimulate further investigations, as well as action to improve the lot of the aged. [75]

A realization of the very complex network of physical, social, and biological factors will increase the understanding of a specific environment: the aged person—patient and/or resident—in nursing homes.

NOTES

1. John D. O'Donahue, "Developing a Conceptual Framework for Planning," Hospital Administration, Fall 1969, pp. 35-54.

2. Erving Goffman, "On the Characteristics of Total Institutions," in Asylums (Garden City, N.Y.: Anchor Books, Doubleday, 1961), pp. 3-124.

3. John Madge, "Aging and the Field of Architecture and Planning," in Aging and the Professions, ed. M. W. Riley, J. W. Riley, Jr., and M. Johnson and Associates (New York: Basic Books and Russell Sage Foundation, 1969).

4. Ibid.

5. National Center for Health Statistics, Health Services and Mental Health Administration, Institutions for the Aged and Chronically Ill: United States, April-June 1963, Vital and Health Statistics, Series 12, no. 1, Department of Health, Education and Welfare Publication no. 1000 (Washington, D.C.: U.S. Government Printing Office, July 1965).

6. Percentage breakdowns are taken from National Center for Health Statistics, Health Services and Mental Health Administration, Selected Characteristics of Nursing Homes for the Aged and Chronically Ill: United States, June-August 1964, Vital and Health Statistics, Series 12, no. 23, Department of Health, Education and Welfare Publication no. 74-1708 (Washington, D.C.: U.S. Government Printing Office, January 1974).

7. National Center for Health Statistics, Health Services and Mental Health Administration, Selected Operating and Financial Characteristics of Nursing Homes: United States, 1973-74, Vital and

Health Statistics, Series 13, no. 22, Department of Health, Education and Welfare Publication no (HRA) 76-1773 (Washington, D.C.: U.S. Government Printing Office, December 1975).

8. U.S. Department of Health, Education and Welfare, Social Security Administration, Conditions of Participation for Extended Care Facilities: Health Insurance for the Aged (Washington, D.C.: Government Printing Office, 1966).

9. National Center for Health Statistics, Selected Operating and Financial Characteristics of Nursing Homes.

10. U.S. Department of Health, Education and Welfare, Your Medicare Handbook, Publication no. (SSA) 74-10050 (Washington, D.C.: Government Printing Office, August 1974).

11. U.S. Office of Human Development, Administration on Aging, Technical assistance memorandum, October 30, 1975.

12. Dorothea Jaeger and Leo W. Simmons, The Aged Ill: Coping with Problems in Geriatric Care (New York: Appleton-Century-Crofts, 1970).

13. Charles J. Karcher and Leonard L. Linden, "Family Rejection of the Aged in Nursing Homes," International Journal of Aging and Human Development 5 (1974): 231-44.

14. Goffman, "On the Characteristics of Total Institutions."

15. James O. Hepner and Donna M. Hepner, The Health Strategy Game (St. Louis: C. V. Mosby, 1973).

16. U.S. Department of Health, Education and Welfare, Your Medicare Handbook; What Is Medicaid?, mimeographed memo to Department of Human Resources staff (1975); U.S. Congress, Senate, Special Committee on Aging, Subcommittee on Long Term Care, Introductory Report: Nursing Home Care in the United States: Failure in Public Policy, 93d Cong., 2d sess.

17. U.S. Department of Health, Education and Welfare, Social and Rehabilitation Services, Medicaid, Medicare: Which Is Which?, Publication no. (SRS) 75-24902 (Washington, D.C.: Government Printing Office, July 1975).

18. U.S. Congress, Senate, Special Committee on Aging, Subcommittee on Long Term Care, Introductory Report.

19. U.S. Congress, Senate, Congressional Record, 93d Cong., 2d sess., 1974, 120, pt. 163.

20. U.S. Congress, Senate, Special Committee on Aging, Subcommittee on Long Term Care, Introductory Report.

21. U.S. Congress, Senate, Special Committee on Aging, Subcommittee on Long Term Care, Supporting Paper No. 1: The Litany of Nursing Home Abuses and an Examination of the Roots of Controversy, 93d Cong., 2d sess., December 1974.

22. U.S. Congress, Senate, Special Committee on Aging, Subcommittee on Long Term Care, Supporting Paper No. 2: Drugs in Nursing Homes: Misuse, High Cost, and Kickbacks, 94th Cong., 1st sess., January 1975.

23. U.S. Congress, Senate, Special Committee on Aging, Subcommittee on Long Term Care, Supporting Paper No. 3: Doctors in Nursing Homes: The Shunned Responsibility, 94th Cong., 1st sess., February 1975.

24. U.S. Congress, Senate, Special Committee on Aging, Subcommittee on Long Term Care, Supporting Paper No. 4: Nurses in Nursing Homes: The Heavy Burden, 94th Cong., 1st sess., April 1975.

25. U.S. Congress, Senate, Special Committee on Aging, Subcommittee on Long Term Care, Supporting Paper No. 5: The Continuing Chronicle of Nursing Home Fires, 94th Cong., 1st sess., August 1975.

26. U.S. Congress, Senate, Special Committee on Aging, Subcommittee on Long Term Care, Supporting Paper No. 6: What Can Be Done in Nursing Homes: Positive Aspects in Long Term Care, 94th Cong., 1st sess., September 1975.

27. Ibid.

28. U.S. Congress, Senate, Special Committee on Aging, Subcommittee on Long Term Care, Supporting Paper No. 7: The Role of Nursing Homes in Caring for Discharged Mental Patients (and the Birth of a For-Profit Boarding Home Industry), 94th Cong., 1st sess., March 1975.

29. U.S. Congress, Senate, Special Committee on Aging, Subcommittee on Long Term Care, Supporting Paper No. 6.

30. Ibid.

31. American Nurses Association, Committee on Skilled Nursing Care, Nursing and Long Term Care: Toward Quality Care for the Aging (American Nurses Association, 1975).

32. U.S. Public Law 93-641, National Health Planning Resources and Development Act of 1974.

33. Elaine B. von Rosenstial, "Criteria and Standards for Institutional Long Term Care," mimeographed (Seattle: University of Washington, Health Services Criteria Project, December 1975).

34. Anselm L. Strauss, Chronic Illness and the Quality of Life (St. Louis: C. V. Mosby, 1975).

35. National Center for Health Statistics, Health Services and Mental Health Administration, Employees in Nursing Homes: United States, April-September 1968, Vital and Health Statistics, Series 12, no. 15, Department of Health, Education and Welfare Publication no. (HSM) 73-1700 (Washington, D.C.: U.S. Government Printing Office, October 1972).

36. National Center for Health Statistics, Health Services and Mental Health Administration, Administrators of Nursing and Personal Care Homes: United States, June–August 1969, Vital and Health Statistics, Series 12, no. 20, Department of Health, Education and Welfare Publication no. (HSM) 73-1705 (Washington, D.C.: U.S. Government Printing Office, March 1973).

37. State of Washington, Legislature, Rules and Regulations of the Board of Examiners for Licensing of Nursing Home Administrators of the State of Washington, 41st sess., 1970.

38. Ilse J. Volinn, "Nursing Home Administrators Licensed in Washington," mimeographed (Olympia: Washington State Department of Social and Health Services, October 1971).

39. American Nurses Association, "Report of the National Conference for Nursing Home Administrators and Directors" (paper presented at National Conference for Nursing Home Administrators and Directors, August 1-2, 1974).

40. American Nurses Association, Committee on Skilled Nursing Care, Nursing and Long Term Care.

41. Ilse J. Volinn, "Professional Nurses in Washington State. A Comparison: 1970-1969-1961-1957," mimeographed (Olympia: Washington State Department of Social and Health Services, June 1971).

42. Ibid.

43. Doris R. Schwartz, "Aging and the Field of Nursing," in Aging and the Professions, pp. 79-113.

44. National Center for Health Statistics, Employees in Nursing Homes.

45. Ilse J. Volinn, "Practical Nurses Licensed in Washington State," mimeographed (Olympia: Washington State Department of Social and Health Services, November 1969).

46. Peter Townsend, Old Age: The Last Segregation (New York: Grossman, 1971).

47. Jaber F. Gubrium and Margaret Ksander, "On Multiple Realities and Reality Orientation," The Gerontologist 15 (1975): 142-45.

48. National Center for Health Statistics, Health Services and Mental Health Administration, Measures of Chronic Illness Among Residents of Nursing and Personal Care Homes: United States, June–August 1969, Vital and Health Statistics, Series 12, no. 24, Department of Health, Education and Welfare Publication no (HRA) 74-1704.

49. U.S. Department of Commerce, Bureau of the Census, Census Population, 1970: Detailed Characteristics, Final Report PC (1) D1, U.S. Summary (Washington, D.C.: U.S. Government Printing Office, 1973).

50. National Center for Health Statistics, Health in the Later Years of Life (Rockville, Md.: U.S. Department of Health, Education and Welfare, Public Health Service, Mental Health Administration, October 1971).

51. National Center for Health Statistics, Health Services and Mental Health Administration, Characteristics of Residents in Nursing and Personal Care Homes: United States, June–August 1964, Vital and Health Statistics, Series 12, no. 19, Department of Health, Education and Welfare Publication no. (HSM) 73-1704 (Washington, D.C.: U.S. Government Printing Office, February 1973).

52. National Center for Health Statistics, Health Services and Mental Health Administration, Measures of Chronic Illness Among Residents of Nursing and Personal Care Homes.

53. L. Mayo, "Problem and Challenge," in Guides to Action on Chronic Illness (New York: National Health Council, 1956), pp. 9-13, 35, 55.

54. Strauss, Chronic Illness and the Quality of Life.

55. Ibid.

56. Jess B. Spielholz and Ilse J. Volinn, "Comparison Study of Convalescent Hospitals and Other Health Facilities," mimeographed (Olympia: Washington State Department of Health, February 1968).

57. Barney G. Glaser and Anselm L. Strauss, Status Passage: A Formal Theory (Chicago: Aldine-Atherton, 1971).

58. Ibid.

59. Jaber F. Gubrium, "Death Worlds in a Nursing Home," Urban Life 4 (1975): 317-38.

60. Goffman, "On the Characteristics of Total Institutions."

61. Gubrium, "Death Worlds in a Nursing Home."

62. Victor W. Marshall, "Organizational Features of Terminal Status Passage in Residential Facilities for the Aged," Urban Life 4 (1975): 349-68.

63. R. Sommer, Personal Space: The Behavioral Basis of Design (Englewood Cliffs, N.J.: Prentice-Hall, 1969).

64. J. Weinberg, "Environment, Its Language and the Aging," Journal of the American Geriatric Society 18 (1970): 681-86.

65. Lynn E. McClannahan, "Therapeutic and Prosthetic Living Arrangements for Nursing Home Residents," The Gerontologist 13 (1973): 424-29.

66. Madge, "Aging and the Field of Architecture and Planning."

67. L. A. Pastalan and D. H. Carson, "Spatial Behavior of Older People," mimeographed (Ann Arbor: Wayne State University-University of Michigan, Institute of Gerontology, 1970).

68. Dean C. Jones, "Spatial Proximity, Interpersonal Conflict and Friendship Formation in the Intermediate Care Facility," The Gerontologist 15 (1975): 150-54.

69. Von Rosenstial, "Criteria and Standards for Institutional Long Term Care."

70. Townsend, Old Age.

71. Robert N. Butler, "Public Interest Report No. 13: The Nursing Home Cover-Up," International Journal of Aging and Human Development 5 (1974): 295-97.

72. Robert N. Butler, "Public Interest Report No. 15: Is There an Ideal Form of Care of the Old?" International Journal of Aging and Human Development 6 (1975): 75-76.

73. National Consumer League, New Help for the Consumer (Washington, D.C., 1974).

74. U.S. Department of Health, Education and Welfare, Public Health Service, Office of Nursing Home Affairs, Long Term Care Facility Improvement Study: Introductory Report (Washington, D.C.: Government Printing Office, July 1975).

75. Ilse J. Volinn, "Gerontological Research and Public Health," Public Health Reviews 3 (1974): 73-90.

APPENDIX
METHODOLOGY OF
CANADIAN SURVEY

MANAGER SURVEY

This survey was one part of a nationwide Canadian study of non-nursing home subsidized housing for the elderly completed in 1973; the other parts were a survey of elderly residents and 19 case studies. The study was conducted by the Canadian Council for Social Development, with the author as chief investigator. The Canadian equivalent of HUD, the Central Mortgage and Housing Corporation (CMHC) financed it. The data were collected in 1971-72. The author took part in all stages of the work. She designed the questionnaire, chose the sample with the assistance of William Nicholls of the University of California Survey Research Center at Berkeley, and CCSD staff. She directed the pretests, worked on the code book, directed coding and data processing, supervised table construction, and did the analysis and wrote the report. She did likewise on the user study, but, there, most of the interviewing was done by assistants, though she visited several developments. She did three of the case studies in this book and supervised the fourth, done by Doug Halverson, and later collected additional data on this one, Summerset Court.

Sample Selection

The sampling frame consisted of a list of developments for the elderly financed by the CMHC and the Canadian National Housing Act (NHA) sections 16, 16A, 35A, and 35D. The list was compiled after a complete review of CHMC loan and public housing files. Nursing homes were as far as possible excluded.

The universe of all NHA developments for the elderly was first stratified by province. To achieve meaningful national results as well as valid figures for each region of the country, a 100 percent sample was selected in provinces with fewer than 60 developments. This meant that questionnaires were sent to all developments in Newfoundland, Prince Edward Island, Nova Scotia, New Brunswick, and Alberta.

For the remaining five provinces, the list of developments in the universe was then stratified by community size (metropolitan and nonmetropolitan, according to census criteria). In the nonmetropolitan areas of each of these provinces, cluster sampling was used; the developments were first clustered geographically by census areas into groups of about 8 to 12 developments, and then one-third of the clusters were randomly selected. Within each of the selected clusters all developments were sampled. This method was used after consultation with Nicholls.

In the metropolitan areas of provinces in which the universe was not sampled, developments were further stratified by sponsor type (public and nonprofit); and the public housing developments were further stratified according to whether the site housed old people only or mixed with families (in different buildings). All metropolitan developments were further stratified by accommodation type (self-contained, congregate, and mixed), and development size (1-20 units/ beds, 21-40, 41-80, 81-149, and 150 or over). Then, a uniform sampling fraction of 50 percent was used, which meant that one-half of the developments in each of the strata were randomly sampled.

In order to achieve as high a return rate as possible, two followup letters were sent after the initial mailing to nonprofit developments, followed by a final telegram. Questionnaires for completion by public housing authorities were channeled through provincial housing corporations, who forwarded them with a covering letter to the various authorities in each case; the completed questionnaires were returned directly to the study staff in Ottawa.

Table A.1 outlines the sample selection process. The universe from which the sample was drawn was constructed from CMHC loan approval lists and originally consisted of 882 developments. On the basis of further contact with CMHC regional offices and returned questionnaires, it was found that 80 cases in the original sample were inappropriate; that is, they consisted of duplications, uncompleted and unoccupied developments, family occupied accommodation, and exclusively nursing care accommodation. When these were excluded, the original sample was reduced to 746, and that sample to 313. From the final sample of 313, 294 questionnaires, or 94 percent, were returned and processed. The response rate was 97 percent for nonprofit developments and 88 percent for the public housing sector.

The returned questionnaires were coded and keypunched in Ottawa and the data then sent to the Berkeley Survey Research Center for processing.

The results presented were not weighted to compensate for the different sampling fractions used for the metropolitan and nonmetropolitan areas of each of the five provinces (one-half and one-third). Although in terms of community size the overall national representation is good, it should be remembered in looking at the results that in five provinces, metropolitan developments are overrepresented and nonmetropolitan developments are underrepresented.

TABLE A.1

Sampling Processes

Process	Nonprofit Developments	Public Housing Developments	Developments
Original universe	585	139	882
Original sample	254	139	393
Adjustments			
Duplications in Central Mortgage and Housing Corporation loan records	8	1	9
Developments uncompleted or unoccupied	18	31	49
Occupied by families	—	3	3
Exclusively nursing accommodation	12	7	19
	38	42	80
Final universe	530	216	746
Final sample	216	97	313
Questionnaires returned	209	85	294
Response rate (percent)	97	88	94
Returned questionnaires as proportion of final universe (percent)	39	40	39

Source: Canadian manager survey.

Sample Validity

Considering the size of the sample, the high response rate, and the elaborate sampling procedure, the data would be expected to have a high degree of validity. This was, in fact, confirmed by comparing the basic characteristics of the processed sample with characteristics of the universe of NHA housing.

In terms of sponsor type, the sample was identical to the universe. In terms of accommodation type, self-contained developments were slightly overrepresented and congregates slightly underrepresented (by 6 percent). When it came to development size, developments with fewer than 21 units or beds were slightly underrepresented (by 5 percent), and developments with 21-40 were very slightly overrepresented (by 3 percent); the proportion of larger developments was practically identical in the sample and universe.

Regional breakdown was as follows: the Atlantic provinces were somewhat overrepresented in the sample (by 12 percent); the prairies were slightly underrepresented (by 7 percent); for Quebec, Ontario, and British Columbia, differences in the sample and universe were negligible. The overrepresentation in the Atlantic region was due to the high response rate there; this had the effect of slightly deflating the national figures on availability of services and facilities since they were less frequent there than in the rest of Canada.

In terms of community size, metropolitan developments were very slightly overrepresented (by 3 percent) and small towns slightly underrepresented (by 6 percent).

Major Sample Characteristics

This section presents more detailed data on some of the basic characteristics of the processed sample; it provides a further check on sample validity and may be helpful in interpreting certain findings.

Sponsorship

Seventy-one percent of the developments in the sample were operated by nonprofit sponsors and 29 percent were operated by public housing agencies. The public housing was built mainly by provincial housing corporations or under joint federal-provincial arrangements, and usually managed by local housing authorities. Although all the housing in Quebec was managed by nonprofit groups, it was built mostly by the Quebec Housing Corporation. More nonprofit developments were located in the Prairies than in any other region, whereas the public housing developments were concentrated in Ontario.

Looking at the breakdown of developments by sponsor group, of the slightly under two-thirds of the sampled developments from whom we were able to obtain the information, 44 percent were operated by service clubs, 18 percent by provincial government agencies, 14 percent by municipalities, 13 percent by other types of nonprofit organizations (mainly of a local nature), 8 percent by churches, and 3 percent by ethnic groups. Practically all of the provincially operated developments and many of the municipally run ones would be public housing.

All of the public housing developments offered self-contained apartment accommodation only. Of the nonprofit developments, 65 percent offered self-contained accommodation, 21 percent offered congregate accommodation (some of which contained nursing beds), and 31 percent offered a mixture of congregate and self-contained accommodation.

As for the relationship between sponsor type and community size, nonprofit accommodation was concentrated mainly in major small towns and metropolitan areas; this was the case for public housing too, although compared to nonprofit housing, more was found in medium-sized cities (21 percent, compared with 4 percent). The latter can be accounted for by the operations of the Ontario Housing Corporation, which has not built housing developments for the elderly in metropolitan Toronto but distributed them throughout numerous other cities in the province.

As for the relationship between sponsor type and development size, as measured by the number of dwelling units or congregate beds, 28 percent of developments had fewer than 21 units or beds; 23 percent had 21-40 units or beds; 27 percent had 41-80 units or beds; 13 percent had 81-149 units or beds; and 8 percent had 150 or more units or beds. Both public and nonprofit housing tended to be concentrated in developments having 80 or fewer units or beds, but compared with public housing the nonprofit sector had a higher proportion of developments with over 40 units or beds.

USER SURVEY

This sample was chosen from 19 Canadian specially designed elderly developments representing the various types of developments across the country. The study was done by the Canadian Council for Social Development, with the author as chief investigator. Interviewing was done in 1971-72. The size of the user sample selected in each development was proportionate to the size of the development. In all cases, it was sufficiently large (not under 10 percent) to satisfy scientific sampling criteria. The following sampling fractions were used:

Number of Dwelling Units or Congregate Housing Beds in Development	Sample Size (percent)
15	40
15-25	35
26-50	30
51-70	25
71-85	20

Number of Dwelling Units or Congregate Housing Beds in Development	Sample Size (percent)
86–100	15
101–125	12
126–250	10
Over 250	25

In each development, elderly residents were selected for interviews by means of a probability sampling procedure (systematic or quasi-random sampling as opposed to simple random sampling). This was applied to tenant lists (most were alphabetically ordered), which, in the case of mixed developments, had been stratified according to accommodation type (congregate housing beds and dwelling units). In the one or two developments that lacked a tenant list, respondents were selected according to the number of their unit (for example, every fifth or tenth door, depending on the sampling fraction). A total of 303 residents were interviewed.

Interviews were arranged through letters, which also introduced the field worker and explained the purpose of the study. Confidentiality was stressed, and it was made clear that the research staff was not connected with the development's management. In most developments, a very low rate of refusal was encountered. Where a refusal or absence occurred, interviewers were instructed to select another respondent. Also, where it was obvious, after ten minutes of interviewing, that the respondent was very confused or uncomprehending (the interview was constructed to detect this), the interview was ended and another resident was selected instead; this was necessary in only three cases. The four trained interviewers were used; three had a background in sociology and psychology, and one was French speaking.

An interview schedule was used; it contained 81 questions and required the interviewer to record 11 sets of impressions. Some of the questions were open-ended, and interviewers were permitted to rephrase questions if they thought it would help the respondent. In the province of Quebec, interviews were conducted in French, using a French interview schedule. The average interview time was 50 minutes, after pretesting.

Residents' responses were coded and punched on IBM cards in Ottawa. The data were then processed at the Berkeley Survey Research Center.

Sample Validity

Although, in a strict sense, our probability sample is representative only of the 19 developments selected for case study, it appears to correspond well in many respects to the total population of NHA-financed housing for the elderly in Canada. The national representativeness of our sample is indicated by comparison of some of the user data with the known national data on all developments, and also with the data that emerged from our national probability sample of housing managers.

In terms of the distribution of NHA-financed accommodation for the elderly in the various regions of the country, our sample was fairly representative of the Atlantic provinces, the prairies, and British Columbia. Quebec, however, is overrepresented in the user survey, and Ontario is underrepresented.

The user survey overrepresents residents of large urban areas: 73 percent of the respondents lived in metropolitan and major urban areas (census terms), whereas by the end of 1970 only 39 percent of all NHA-financed developments for the elderly were located in metropolitan and major urban areas. However, the bias is not as great as these figures indicate because developments in metropolitan and major urban centers tend to be much larger than those in small towns (and, consequently, larger than the developments in rural areas).

In terms of sponsor type, the user survey sample is fairly representative of the population of NHA housing for the elderly. In the user survey sample, 68 percent of respondents lived in nonprofit developments and 32 percent in public housing; in the total population, 64 percent of all dwelling units and congregate housing beds were built by nonprofit sponsors and 36 percent by public housing agencies.

In terms of accommodation type, the user sample was fairly representative of the national population of NHA-financed housing for the elderly build by the end of 1970. In the user sample, 37 percent of the respondents were in congregate accommodation and 63 percent in self-contained apartments. In the NHA housing, 25 percent of the residents were in congregate accommodation.

Some of the demographic characteristics of the user survey sample can be compared to the national stratified probability sample on which the manager survey that was part of the same study was based, although differences in question wording complicate this task. Nevertheless, it is clear that, in terms of the age range of residents, the user sample corresponds fairly closely to the national sample. In the user study, 60 percent of respondents were aged 75 and older. In the manager survey, only 40 percent of managers said that the largest group in this development was aged 75 and over (reported by 63 percent of hostel managers and 22 percent of the managers of self-contained developments). However, the apparent discrepancy between respondents' ages in the user and manager surveys decreases when one takes into account that congregate developments tend to be much

larger than self-contained apartment developments. On the basis of
further analysis of the statistical universe and the management study
sample, it appears that the user study respondents were probably
slightly older than all residents of NHA-financed housing for the elderly.

When it comes to health status, 78 percent of the user survey
respondents said that they had no health problems, or only slight disabilities, while 64 percent of the manager respondents claimed that
none of their residents had serious health limitations. The questions
in the two surveys differ to such an extent that comparisons are difficult; but it would appear that the prevalence of serious physical incapacities is probably not significantly different between the two samples.

The sex of over two-thirds (69 percent) of the user sample was
female. This appears to be fairly typical of all housing developments.
In the manager survey, only 10 percent of developments reported
one-half or more male residents, 57 percent reported less than a
quarter males, and 32 percent reported one-fourth to one-half males.

The financial status of residents appears to differ in the user
and the management surveys. In the user survey, only 35 percent of
residents said they were dependent solely on the old-age security
pension and guaranteed income supplement; in the manager survey,
however, 69 percent of developments reported that most of their residents were dependent solely on the pension and supplement. This
discrepancy might be explained by managers' lack of awareness of
residents' financial resources, or by the reluctance of user survey
respondents to admit to having no other income.

ELIZABETH D. HUTTMAN is Professor of Sociology at California State University, Hayward. She was previously assistant professor at the University of British Columbia.

Dr. Huttman has done research on social aspects of housing for over 15 years. She was chief investigator for a Canadian nationwide study of housing and social services for the elderly and has taken part in an American nationwide study of the elderly under the housing allowance program. She has coauthored a book on housing the elderly, Beyond Shelter. Her articles have appeared in the Journal for Sociology and Social Welfare, Journal of the American Orthopsychiatric Association, Sociological Symposium, Annals of Regional Science, and The City.

Dr. Huttman holds a B.A. from Syracuse University, an M.Sc. from Cornell University, and a Ph.D. from the University of California, Berkeley.

ILSE J. VOLINN is Clinical Assistant Professor at the School of Physiological Nursing, University of Washington and a private consultant.

Dr. Volinn has done research for the U.S. Public Health Service Region X, the Washington State Department of Social and Health Services, Skid Road Community Council, and the University of Washington's School of Social Work. She was also a research project director for the federally funded Health Manpower Project and health research specialist for the Washington State Hospital Commission. She wrote "A Comparison Study of Convalescent Hospitals and Other Health Facilities" for the Washington State Department of Social and Health Services. Her articles have appeared in Public Health Reviews and Health Reports.

Dr. Volinn holds a Ph.D. in philology from the University of Vienna, Austria, and an M.A. in Sociology from the University of Washington, Seattle.